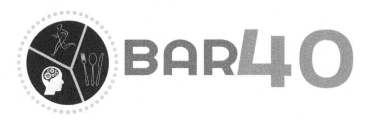

Achieving Personal Excellence

2021 Edition

Your Ultimate 52-Week Training Resource
for Reaching Peak Potential

Eric J. Bartosz

BAR40 Achieving Personal Excellence - Your Ultimate 52-Week Training Resource for Reaching Peak Potential rev. by Eric Bartosz
Copyright © 2021

Project managed with AuthorDock.com

ISBN: 978-1629671819

Library of Congress Control Number: 2020913612

Any references to historical events, real people or real places are used fictitiously. Names, characters, and places are products of the author's imagination.

Front cover image by Cole Marie Designs

www.bar40.org

Reader Reviews of BAR40

Transform Now !!!

What I loved immediately about Eric's book is his own experiences that he shares in an intimate way that so many others forgo. Eric's ability to "pull back the curtain" on his own process is shared throughout the book. This lends an access point that, for myself, seems to create a level of ease and "I can do this" feeling that is a first for me when reading anything like this before. A true gift!

I highly recommend this book to anyone who is looking for true transformation. I would also recommend this book to anyone who is thinking of writing books like this or looking how to approach others when introducing new ideas and systems, processes to help improve your life! Many self-help gurus can learn something by studying Eric's approach, style and dynamic mind set(s).

— KB

The Enthusiasm Jumps off the Page!

As soon as you begin reading, Eric's excitement and enthusiasm pull you in. He's clearly devoted his energy and time to helping others achieve personal excellence.

I've never seen anyone distill the pieces of excellence down to such an easy to understand framework as Eric has done with mindset, diet, and fitness. Eric walks you through how to gain control of each of these pieces and where to point them to be the best version of you.

The included journal was also a nice touch. It's easy to get distracted when tapping into our digital lives for calendars, journals, etc. and this physical copy keeps you focused and on track for the full 52 week program!

Highly recommend it to anyone who is ready to put in the hard work to truly improve themselves.

— JMM

Love it so far!

I feel like I'm sitting down with a friend and making some great future goals. I read quite a bit for work and don't have time to read something like this often, and now I know why. I guess I feel too busy, but the reality is I haven't made it a goal and I haven't invested the time in developing it as a habit. Love how easy the author pulls his ideas together and makes the book your daily tool for success!

— MH

Motivational - Be the best You

If you're looking for inspiration, and motivation, look no further. Eric is succinct and easy to understand. The daily journal included is a practical tool.

— JA

Great tool to push yourself!!!

This book is such a great resource to push yourself (physically and mentally) through this thing called life. I'm stoked to continue through this program and hit my goals.

I LOVE the daily notes section—totally helps break down the bigger goals and make them attainable. Highly recommend.

— EH

Great read!

The author is a great storyteller and motivator by combining personal experiences and knowledge learned over the years to create a program that can be utilized by just about anyone wanting to make self-improvements in physical and mental health. A must read!

— AR

A Game Changer

This book lays out the foundation for really changing your lifestyle. This year has been tough on everyone and I for one have let myself go. But after reading this book, I have a new set of goals and will work towards a new me. The journal in this book really helps keep track of everything too!

— LA

Great Motivational Read!

A great tool for challenging yourself to your full potential! The program really is an all-around life improving challenge incorporating aspects of physical and mental health unlike many other "similar style" books I've read. I look forward to continuing the program and seeing where it takes me.

— BR

BAR40 here I come for my best year ever!

BAR40 has helped me to tweak some of my daily decisions allowing me to make better choices. Unlike other books that I've read, I'm not done with this one now that I've read it. The author, Eric Bartosz, has provided me with my first ever log to track my daily progress. He has also shared some additional works that are of interest and sound like they complement BAR40 nicely. I will be keeping BAR40 on my nightstand! Overall BAR40 has left me with the feeling that I have a friend beside me as I travel along this journey towards having the best year ever! I am recommending BAR40 to people of any fitness level as you work towards a better version of yourself.

— MM

BAR40 can be transformative for those who truly desire positive change in their lives

Eric has filled the book with useful tools and strategies that can help readers build a customized 1-year plan to reach their peak potential in all the core aspects of their life. His work is based on Eric's own life and years of experience helping others reach their peak potential. The book is structured in a way that uses one's individual goals, preferences, fitness levels and ideas of what success means as starting points. The end result of following BAR40 helps the reader deal with individual habits in a healthier way through the creation of a "self-guided" journey that incorporates universal principles known to enhance personal success. The book's weekly training journal touches on relevant topics such as diet, fitness, daily tools for successes, sobriety, etc. I believe that Eric's brand of life strategy coaching should be a taught in schools starting at a young age since it motivates individuals of all ages to make each waking day matter in a more meaningful way.

— FR

Inspirational, AND pragmatic

What drew me to this book was how it recognizes that each person's goals and abilities are different and focuses on what each person can do to become his/her personal best self. BAR40 met me where I was and has helped me take it up a notch over the last month or so I've been digesting it. Up a notch athletically, but also in terms of my overall attitude. It offers wisdom on how to look at today from future self, focus on realistic goal-setting, and achievement. BAR40 also has good mix of science and some "motherly" kinds of advice on alcohol use and other daily decisions which has made me more thoughtful about choices. One month in, and still using the simple tables and daily notes—which are somehow stickier to use than my fancy Apple watch. The reading list to other authors is also a real nice resource I plan to tap.

— DC

Powerful program for creating consistent results

This book provides a terrific roadmap for creating consistent results in multiple areas of life—the end goal being that of achieving personal excellence. We generally don't end up achieving personal excellence by accident, and even with a great deal of intention, we can still miss the mark. What makes this book unique is the combination of up front coaching /

education combined with the accountability built into the book. Plus, I love the recommended reading. This is a powerful tool for consistently showing up for yourself, setting daily goals and action plans, and following through to observing and noting results. If we can be even just SLIGHTLY better than we were yesterday, we are on our way to creating dramatic results over time. And this book helps people get there.

— HC

BAR40 is the book you need to initiate and sustain positive health and lifestyle choices!

I loved everything about this great, well-articulated, easy to relate to journey the author Eric created to improve his overall health and lifestyle choices! His thought process and life experiences make this the perfect read for anyone seeking some modifications in areas of their everyday living! I highly recommend it, the tracking journal which is included will prove to be priceless!

— DB

For Riley

May each of your years be the best ever.

Table of Contents

Goodbye 2020 and Hello 2021!

My original plan back in January was to write a year in review summary of some of the main headlines that defined 2020. This plan, like so many others, was canceled due to Covid (or Covancelled as the expression goes.) Here's my thinking: I'm writing this 2021 update in late November which means that we have all been living the last eight months of our lives under the umbrella of Covid-19 and there is not much new information I could share that you have not already heard from the news, social media and daily conversations with all of the people in our lives. We're all in this together and are living the same realities with varying degrees of impact. While some of us have been fortunate to remain relatively unscathed throughout this aside from lifestyle changes, so many others have suffered the ultimate loss of losing a loved one, or in many tragic cases, more than one.

A point of note that I found very validating this year was in regard to all of the feedback I received on how the BAR40 methodology served as a personal resource in making these difficult last months slightly more manageable. BAR40 has been around long before Covid-19 ever made its appearance in our lives, but it happens to be particularly well suited for these times. One of the most common conversations I have with people is in regard to how routines have been upended, schedules dismantled, social events canceled and so many uncertainties in life—there has been a continuous current of stress and anxiety in their life. BAR40 is a resource that provides the tools to bring back structure to our daily routine in the form of taking control of the things we can manage without having external forces derail our intents. Specifically, creating an improved diet plan, building a custom fitness regimen that is designed around your schedule and interests, a plan for goal-setting (and achieving!), habit formation/elimination strategies, a suggested reading list of best in class books (each one has the potential to fundamentally improve your life), and using the 52-week daily journal as a personal accountability tool that ties it all together. In the midst of all of the upheaval and turbulence, BAR40 can serve as not only a highly effective field guide toward living your best year ever but it also provides a level of psychological comfort in regaining ownership of core areas.

Also of note in 2020, a very interesting breakthrough test was introduced by Genomind in June of this year called the Mental Health Map. I want to bring this to your attention as it relates to pursuing the best version of yourself through an in-depth understanding of genetic predispositions. As a broad overview, the test is conducted at home with a cheek swab which is returned to Genomind for lab analysis. If you're familiar with the 23andMe test this part may be familiar to you. The rest of the process is completely unique though. Genomind has pioneered the technology to utilize your returned sample to analyze 38 genetic variants and their influence on 29 mental health traits. The results are compiled in a detailed report that you access online and broken down into seven categories including Stress and Anxiety, Mood, Focus and Memory, Substance Abuse and Habits, Sleep, Social

Behavior, and Eating Behavior. Basically, this is the first test available without a prescription that provides a tremendous amount of data analysis on the traits we are born and hardwired with. Why I thought this test was such a radical innovation is that it shows where natural strengths are as well as the areas we should be on the lookout for needing extra attention in order to optimize behaviors . . . or simply be aware of why we may have certain reactions or perceptions. There are no "good or bad" results in this any more than genetic ancestry reports are providing positive or negative information. It's just the facts based on our individual genetic coding. In other words, a look behind the curtain to the inner workings of how we are uniquely programmed to operate since birth. Along with the test results in each category are interpretations and resources such as how to best put to use our natural predispositions to maximize potential mental health and wellness. I'll pause here to say that in no way is this any sort of paid endorsement for Genomind, I mention it based on my personal experience as I took the test a few months ago and was blown away by the results and how much insight the test provided based on that cheek swab. By no means was it 100% accurate but that's not the claim Genomind is making. Simply having a genetic predisposition for a certain tendency or behavior type does not mean that is your destiny in life. Our unique life experiences and the environment will always play a huge role in our personality and perspectives in life along with genetics but having this extra insight provides a lot of pieces to our individual puzzle that was out of reach before this test became available.

So much of our life is defined by our mindset and the lens

through which we perceive the events transpiring around us every day. More than ever the significance of this reality is evident as it relates to our mental grit and resilience in the face of our collective relentless exposure to unsettling news, both political and pandemic related. In looking at this situation with an eye out for opportunity, this reality provides an unmatched opportunity for us to train for mental toughness and practice perseverance. Consider the similarities between 2020 and a prolonged fitness event: there's an old expression that you run the first half of a marathon with your body and the second half with your mind.

In a lot of ways, life during Covid has similarities to an athletic endurance event in that it's pushing many of us way past our normal comfort levels. Instead of our physical boundaries being tested and strained we're now getting into long-range mental mileage territory with the daily stress and constant uncertainty that the last eight months have brought on.

Try taking a page out of the endurance athletes' playbook and use a mindset strategy that takes the finish line out of the equation. When you're at mile 19 of a 26-mile race and starting to feel like you may not make it, the last thing you want to do is dwell on the fact that you have seven more miles. Instead, you're setting small achievable goals on your very short-term horizon to create these micro-successes on your way to the finish line. For the marathon runner that may mean concentrating on making it to the next water table or the yellow car parked in the far distance.

For life in Covid, dwelling too much on when vaccines will be available or whether you will be able to go on vacation next summer can make the finish line seem overwhelmingly far off in the distance. Give this a try instead: direct your focus to set some small goals and priorities over the next few weeks that are both meaningful and achievable. Here's an easy one . . . top 20 list of people you have been meaning to reach out to over the past few months but have not yet gotten around to. Make that list and call, text, or email all of them 20 within 14 days. If you give yourself 20 minutes of contemplation you could probably come up with a list of ideas of what you would like to concentrate on over the coming months . . . aside from the news!

Life in 2020 is full of uncertainty; we can't do much about that. What we can do is build our mental muscles by directing our focus and attention to all of the things within our control. While you're busy focusing on making the days in front of you the best ever the Covid finish line will keep getting closer! While many topics this (election) year have brought divided opinions, one outlook that most everyone seems to agree with is that 2020 can't be over soon enough, and let's hope 2021 brings an abundance of health, happiness, and prosperity for all of us.

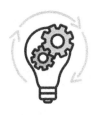

Introduction

Welcome to BAR40! If you're reading this book it's likely for one of a few reasons:

- You've heard about BAR40 from someone who has done it in the past or is currently doing it

- Someone in your life, whether it be family, friend, or co-worker, heard about the program and knew it would be something that you would be interested in doing

- You've checked out our site, videos and/or social media and have decided to make the move and start BAR40

Whatever the case is, I want to be one of the first to say congratulations on beginning what will be a challenging, but fundamentally life-changing experience that will ultimately stay with you long after you have completed the 52-week session.

So what's it all about, and how does it work, you ask? Great questions that will be answered in detail, but as a summary description: BAR40 is a 52-week program equally focused on mind and body that is designed to let you become the best version of yourself and deliver an end result of your personal best year ever.

There are three main elements to BAR40 that are all very much linked together and impact virtually every aspect of our day.

- **Mindset** — This is the commitment to approaching each day with the goal of reaching its full potential, being mindful of making the right choice instead of the easy one, and developing the habit to continuously think in terms of what would your ideal future self do in any particular moment. When you get down to it, the best year ever does not happen at once and is really a collection of best days. BAR40 means developing the habit of relentless pursuit of personal excellence in all aspects of your life and increasing your level of personal accountability to ensure your goals are achieved.

- **Diet** — This is not meant in the traditional sense of "I'm on a diet." BAR40 provides the time where you evaluate the choices you make on what fuel you are putting in your body, how substitutes can be used, and identifying what food/drink habits we have arrived at over the years that should be changed.

- **Exercise** — Without question, BAR40 is a program heavily reliant on physical fitness. Of course, this means planning a program that is safe and suitable for your particular situation, but this component means that exercise will be a significant part of your life for the next 52 weeks. The original BAR40 was geared exclusively toward running and bodyweight exercises, and if that's what you want to go with, I have no doubt you will be amazed at the results. If running is not your thing, there are plenty of substitute options, but the main takeaway is that working out will become a core component of your lifestyle for the next year.

In addition to the mindset, diet, and exercise components, there is also a "1-year sober" challenge, which eliminates alcohol for the 52 weeks. Your first reaction to that may be, Whoa, say what!? I didn't sign up for the no drinking part!" Although the original BAR40 does include getting rid of booze for a year, I do realize that's a commitment some people are just not comfortable making. So while I highly recommended it and will get into the reasoning why in the Drinking section, it's not a deal-breaker if you decide to forego the sobriety aspect of BAR40 . . . but do yourself a favor and keep an open mind about it for the moment! Before we get too far down the road on particulars and specifics, I'll provide some background on the origins of BAR40 to shed some light on the original concept and the many applications it has within our daily lives. First off, the name BAR40 comes from my name, "Bartosz," and when it was started . . . my 40th birthday. It represents the beginning of a journey toward your best year and a turning point in your life that will have permanent results. More on that below . . .

For as long as I can remember, I've had a curiosity and a passion related to the pursuit of continuous personal improvement and the best ways to go about living the best possible life. As we have probably all experienced in some form or another, the greatest intentions and plans can quickly and easily be derailed when some unexpected development in life gets in our way, and we lose sight of what it is we originally set out to do. Whether this is related to diet, career, school, relationships, finance, fitness . . . whatever the case may be . . . the outcome of falling short of a goal can be a mix of disappointment and frustration, not to mention the thing we set out to do didn't get done!

This was on my mind one night when I was at a bar with friends having a conversation about what each of us was planning to do to celebrate our 40th birthday or in a few cases for those already over the 40 threshold, what they had done to commemorate the occasion. As you would expect, all sorts of fun ideas were being thrown around: a huge party, the gambling trip to Vegas, skydiving, a NYC bar crawl, golf at Pebble Beach, skiing in Colorado, a day racing cars, wine tasting in Italy . . . any one of them sounded like a blast! The one common thread that all of these had in common was the fact that they were all an experience-based celebration that was basically a weekend party. Not that there's anything wrong with that, of course. I'd be first in line to happily sign on for any and all of those excursions. More to the point of why I wasn't drawn to that sort of concept was what I had in the back of my mind . . . an unformed but definitely present idea to make my 40th be something that would stand the test of time as a pivotal point in my life and one where the memory rose to the occasion of the milestone. That said, I don't consider 40 to be the major (often dreaded) life event that it's sometimes made out to be, but I did recognize it as the unofficial starting line of our middle age decade and worthy of special consideration.

What came from this line of thinking was the notion of celebrating my 40th not with a birthday blowout weekend but instead making it a tribute that would last until I turned 41 . . . or, simply put, my best year ever. (I'd put my body through quite a bit in the past 40 years, so I figured special thanks were in order!) At this point, I was excited about the concept of pursuing this great year, but what exactly does that mean? As the saying goes: a goal without a plan is just a wish. I decided the best approach would be to isolate and examine various aspects of daily life to make for a more manageable approach toward coming up with an overall plan. This separation process ultimately led to the creation of the core areas that BAR40 zeroes in on: diet, fitness, mindset, and the act of goal setting that ties everything together.

A critical consideration would be sustainability; it had to be something I could do anywhere my work travels took me.

A couple of things are worth mentioning about the one-year duration of BAR40. Your first thought may be that it's too long, after all . . . 52 weeks is a while! Part of the logic behind the one-year commitment is the simple reason that it provides a realistic runway of time to plan, pursue and ultimately achieve the three goals that you have set out to do during BAR40. Of course, different goals will require varying amounts of time, but in the interest of realistic expectations, one year is a length of time that tends to be the right amount for most of what we are setting out to do. Exceptions will always exist, of course, if your goal is to get a certification or degree that is a multi-year endeavor; then, obviously, it's not going to be done in one year. So the goal, in this case, would be taking the initial steps of identifying the program, enrolling, and beginning the process. At the end of the year, your successful achievement will be that you are finally on the path that will ultimately lead to the completion of your sought-after certificate, degree, diploma, etc.

Another aspect of the one year that makes it work so well is in relation to the creation of habits. I can't emphasize enough how fundamental habits are in all our lives and how significant a role they play in our daily lives. (According to a research paper published by Duke University, up to 40% of our daily actions are not decisions at all but habits being executed.) Habits are not inherently good or bad, but simply routines that we have, over time, programmed ourselves to perform. If we think of our subconscious as a super-computer of sorts, it is excellent at identifying ways to become highly efficient at understanding what needs to be done and automatically doing it, thereby freeing up our conscious mind to focus on other tasks. Habits are part of each of our unique computer operating systems.

An easy everyday example would be brushing our teeth. We don't give any specific thought to the process in the sense of "upper right, lower right, upper left, lower left," etc., we just do it without any real thought. You may be able to relate to the times when we are on autopilot to the extent we don't even recall if we brushed at all! There is no shortage of examples of these routines that largely govern our lives every day, and the first step toward meaningful, long-term change is identifying the ones we want to work on eliminating, improving, or implementing.

Our mind and the countless functions that the conscious and subconscious are constantly performing is truly an awesome system. Recent brain imaging technology that has been developed is now allowing us to learn a tremendous amount of new information about what is going on behind the scenes in these brains of ours, but the bottom line is that habits are by no means destiny. Once we understand some basics about how our whole habit system operates, we are able to use that knowledge for amazing, life-changing results.

Because habits are not formed or broken overnight, we need time to successfully create or change them. This is another reason why one year is such an important component of BAR40 and one of the distinguishing factors that will make it so effective for you. Committing to this extended duration is critical to not only achieve fitness results, but also to ensure the new habits have sufficient time to become permanent routines. We do not have to search far to find an opposite example of what does not work. Mass-marketed diet plans are an easy category to look at as typically over 50% of US adults plan to lose weight (about 40% of Americans are now obese, according to the CDC). This industry has a seemingly endless list of options for short term (fad or crash) diets that promise radical weight loss in a few quick weeks or months. Statistically ... these plans simply do not work. As you would expect, there's a tremendous amount of research and reporting available on the typical outcomes of these diets. I won't bore you with a laundry list of them but here are a few interesting ones:

- 65% of people who complete a "fad diet" will end up gaining all the weight back (a fad diet being defined as a diet that is popular for a time without being a standard dietary recommendation)

- 25% of fad dieters will give up the plan within two weeks

- On average, fad dieters will try four different plans each year

A common thread in these plans and the resulting failure is that the underlying habits are not changed. When the brief diet plan is complete, the old habits kick back in . . . or to use the earlier computer example, our default "operating system" runs our standard program again. BAR40 is essentially a framework of habits that collectively work together to improve every aspect of your life that you seek out to change and improve. BAR40 has the tagline of "Best Year Ever," and the best year ever is broken down into 52 best weeks, which of course, is 365 best days. Beginning this practice of looking at each day through the lens of "how do I make today really count" is a small, but mighty change element in how we see and engage with the world around us, and the foundation of the BAR40 program.

BAR40, in its most effective form, is a mindset, a way of reframing our perspective on any and all aspects of our daily actions and behaviors, to question whether our approach is in alignment with living our best year ever. I fully realize this practice of being mindful and "present in the present" is something that may feel completely foreign at first. Let's face it, often the default daily routine is a blur of getting out of bed, getting everyone out the door to work and school, checking off all the to-do list boxes of the day and at some point getting back into bed to get some sleep before we wake up and do it again. While there aren't necessarily individual aspects of this way of living that can be identified as "wrong," it does not lend itself to be our best selves. With this scenario, life can become a repeating habit loop that often spans the years and leaves us shaking our heads and asking, "where does the time go?" As the saying goes, life is what happens when you're busy making plans. If we consider the fact that these habits and behaviors have had extensive periods of time to take root, it's easy to see why it's not an overnight process to change them. But the critical bottom line is that they most certainly *can* be changed ... as you will see for yourself in the coming year.

It would be easy to fill plenty of pages talking about habit, as it is a core component of the success of the BAR40 pro-gram, but a much more valuable exercise is to read (or listen to the audio version of) *The Power of Habit* by Charles Duhigg. This will be the first of monthly reading assignments (more on that topic shortly) and a fantastic deep dive into the study of habits. The book is as entertaining as it is useful in understanding the three universal components to every habit (cue-routine-reward) and how to harness the forces at work in our subconscious and direct them toward achieving our goals. I say with confidence and personal experience that the process of forming new habits is in and of itself habit forming! If you've ever bought a new cooking appliance like an Instapot or air fryer and started looking for new meals to prepare with them, or have gotten a new power-washer and started noticing all the things that could be cleaned up after a good blasting with a high-pressure water stream ... there's a similar, slightly addictive mentality that sets in with creating habits. (You'll have to take my word for it at first, but you'll see for yourself soon enough.)

To get back to the original question of how BAR40 works: the fundamental components are dietary modifications, mindfulness, exercise, goal setting, and alcohol avoidance. (I know that the drinking part makes a lot of people nervous, but no worries. I'll cover that topic in the Drinking chapter and answer all questions.)

This BAR40 book is a tool that you will be using daily for the next 52 weeks to "keep the trains running on time." My hope is that it will become a valued resource in not only recording your successes and progress but that it also serves to keep you on track and moving toward your goals. In our 2021 digital world, some concepts still work best in their analog form, and this book is modeled after the same running and fitness training journal that I've been using for years. In my experience, part of the effectiveness of the book is its constant, tangible presence on my desk, which serves as a very effective and constant reminder to be the best version of myself.

In addition to the fitness log component of the book are the added aspects of the journal. The design is meant to be an all-inclusive unit as opposed to separate books for various aspects of your life. Considering how the collective components and focuses of our daily efforts all interact and overlap, the most effective "capture method" is to keep everything in one place where it's easily reviewed. One of the critical functions of using this physical book as opposed to an online version or app is that it serves as a cue in the habit loop process. As you will read all about in *The Power of Habit*, the cue is what triggers the routine which will ultimately lead to formation of the habits . . . and of course, the habits are a big ingredient in the fuel that is propelling us toward our goals. The simple daily act of recording what went right or wrong, notes on exercise, mileage ran or biked (if applicable), highlights of the day, what we appreciated most and aspects of the day that we wish we had a do-over on . . . these are all aspects of our lives, which, when put together, are greater than the sum of their parts. This daily routine is a remarkably effective way of reflecting on each day and provides a chance to have a few minutes of introspection that we don't often make time for in our over-scheduled daily routines. For years I have done this at the end of each day, and it still never ceases to surprise me how powerful a practice this daily retrospection is. Perhaps part of the reason the book is meant for your eyes only is that the knowledge that no one else will be reading your notes lends itself to honest candor and reveals insights you may not have been consciously aware of.

As you'll find in the BAR40 program, it's a loop where each aspect is connected to the others. Aside from serving as the recording device on the BAR40 journey and pseudo-training partner, the main job of the book starting now, on Day 1, is acting as a visual reminder to start asking yourself the question, Is what I'm doing now/today in alignment with how I see the best version of myself? It goes without saying that, for all of us, the answer will sometimes be, "not really." That is of little importance compared to the main objective of creating a default mindset of increased self-awareness and continuous minor course-corrections that keep you oriented and moving toward your set goals.

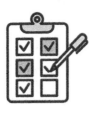

Goals

In my mind, establishing your personal goals is one of the most exciting aspects of BAR40, as these will serve as the framework for your motivation over the next 52 weeks. This step should be given the proper amount of consideration and is worthy of taking the time to reflect upon in case you don't have immediate objectives in mind. One approach is to sit down with a pen and pad and think about it like this: Imagine yourself at a party or out to dinner with a group of friends and the question comes up, Fast answer . . . if you could wave a magic wand and accomplish three life priorities in the next 12 months, what would they be? While there may not be three things that immediately pop into mind, you may get one or two, and that would be a starting point to begin drawing out your most significant goals. Sometimes our immediate response gives voice to our subconscious and can be highly effective at bypassing our conscious thinking.

For a great example of this process in action and a quick method of helping someone with a "one or the other" type of decision, try this the next time you're with someone having a tough time with a choice. Everyone is familiar with the tried and true approach of flipping a coin to come to a decision, so start it off that way assigning heads and tails to the two options. Flip the coin and while it's in the air, ask your indecisive friend, Quick . . . what do you want it to be?! They have, literally, only a second to answer, so their impulsive and immediate response will answer the question they were grappling with on a conscious level, but subconsciously had a clear direction on. (Or you may get a "wait . . . what?" while the coin is spinning in the air and mission not accomplished!) At any rate, give it a try, and you'll see. Unfortunately, it's a bit of a "one per customer" scenario, and that goes for personal use as well. Once the approach is known, the fundamental element of the impulse response is lost.

As a personal example, when I first did BAR40 and thought about what my future self would be most proud of accomplishing, I looked back over the years and tried to identify any bucket list items that I had always wanted to pursue but for whatever reason had not . . . typical "life gets in the way" outcomes that almost all of us can relate to. One of the goals that I arrived at was becoming a firefighter. I was born in Massachusetts, and growing up, my father and grandfather were both career firefighters. I always looked at the role of a first responder as a very meaningful calling, and during my high school years, I gave firefighting or law enforcement serious consideration as a profession. Ultimately, I ended up pursuing a path in business instead, but the drive and instinct to help others never diminished; it simply manifested itself through different channels.

In 1999 I relocated from Massachusetts to New York City, and short of joining the FDNY, my options for becoming involved in the fire service were extremely limited. Ten years later, my wife, Trish, and I moved 90 miles west to Pennsylvania in advance of the birth of our daughter and settled in our new home in the Lehigh Valley. Each state in the US has its own breakdown of how fire departments are structured, but in general, the three categories can be classified as career, volunteer, or a combination. Pennsylvania is predominantly a volunteer state, with 90% of departments falling into the unpaid category, and the fire department was located less than a mile from our house. While I was certainly aware of the proximity of the fire station and the fact that it was a volunteer department, I did not give serious consideration to submitting an application the first years we lived in Pennsylvania based on the universally familiar mentality of "life's too busy now, maybe in the future at some point."

It was only when I took this first goal-setting step of self-analysis and invested the time and effort to envision a more panoramic view of the present and future that true priorities came into focus.

For about a week, I was thinking about goals every day while I ran. Something triggered a memory of my grandfather, and just like that, the realization popped into my head that fire-fighting was a perfect example of an unfulfilled but pending life goal. As quick as that, the idea solidly clicked into place, and I knew with certainty that it was a pursuit I would be passionate about.

For the actual process of selecting goals, there isn't any best time and place aside from whatever works best for you to carve out some part of your day to set aside for (relatively) uninterrupted thought. I mentioned above that for me, it's running. I have always found that if I need to give something any serious consideration, try to figure out a challenge, come up with creative ideas, work on a talk or presentation that I will be giving or anything else that requires some contemplation . . . for me running has always been the optimal time to deliver maximum results. Of course, this isn't just an anecdotal ob-servation as there is plenty of research and data available that has shown exercise, especially cardio, gives a significant brainpower boost via the extra blood being pumped to your brain and the corresponding oxygen and nutrients. (More on that in the Exercise section.) I point it out simply to say that you may find this is the best time to channel your thoughts into the direction of what your Top 3 prioritized goals will be for the next year. Another option is while driving. If your work requires a daily commute, then you may have plenty of experience with rush hour traffic to some extent, or maybe it's just a long ride. Either way, that windshield time becomes routine, and our minds tend to wander so in that sense it's an ideal opportunity to harness your thinking and direct it toward a productive exercise . . . the goal of setting goals!

It's worth mentioning that this process of identifying and establishing goals is geared toward helping you come up with what awesome and meaningful pursuits are most important to you. But perhaps you already know exactly what you would like to dedicate this BAR40 time toward. Great! In either scenario, once you have chosen some goals, a next step is running them through a quick test, like checking a boat for leaks while it's still at the dock instead of 20 miles from shore.

I've always found the SMART acronym to be a simple and effective filter of sorts to determine the likelihood of ultimate success. I first started using this about 20 years ago after spending a semester listening to my professor in a management class beat the drum relentlessly on how this tool should be the final step for any company in decision making, everything from setting its strategic objectives in the marketplace to each department manager sitting down with individual employees during their performance reviews and setting objectives. It's a straightforward way to hold up a goal, give it a shake to see if it holds together and one you have perhaps used before:

S *Specific* — Your goal is focused and has a tangible outcome. If the goal is vague or not well-defined, it will not provide a clear target. For example, a goal of "I want to eat better" is too general and broad for the level of detail needed to lead to a specific result. For this one, you should be able to write down a clear description of what the achievement is.

M *Measurable* — The goal needs to have a clear definition of what success means. This part provides the answer to how success is quantified and also provides a framework for evaluating and tracking progress. Reaching goals typically involves a progression of steps and those can be looked at in relation to the ultimate end but need to have measurable aspects to define where you are in relation to the final achievement. One example may be that you want to run a 5k in less than 30 minutes. Being able to look at individual mile times during your process of getting there is critical to understanding how you are tracking toward the 30-minute target.

A *Achievable* — Is this goal something that can be accomplished with the available time and resources? The goal needs to provide a sufficient challenge but not become unrealistic or impossible. Part of this component can be listing what steps are needed to make the goal happen and identifying potential barriers that would make it impossible. While the goal of taking a selfie in your favorite t-shirt on all seven continents is awesome and may meet the other SMART criteria, unless you have a lot of free time in the next 12 months, it's not achievable, so the goal fails the test. (If you do have the circumstances to take such a globe-trotting adventure, more power to you and I'd love to see the photos during your amazing trip!)

R *Relevant* — This is one of the most critical factors, in my opinion. BAR40 is made for helping you achieve your best year ever, and so the pursuits you decide on should reflect what's most important to you. This step also helps ensure the goal is a priority that will keep you motivated throughout the year. There isn't a right or wrong answer for this one as long as it's meaningful to you. A goal of riding your bike three days a week because your spouse keeps bugging you to ride your bike more (but you absolutely hate riding your bike) does not score well on the relevance test. The same exact goal—reframed in the context of you would love to ride your bike three days a week but never make the time for it—makes it very relevant. That's a straightforward example but understanding the motivation and intent of the goals we are considering helps lend some clarity to where it lands on our own personal hierarchy of outcomes.

T *Time-bound* — For BAR40 purposes, this final component is straightforward as the 52-week duration automatically puts a schedule on the goal. One point of note on this would be if the goal you have in mind falls far short of this, then perhaps it's worth considering adding an additional goal. It's entirely possible that there is something on your top priority life's to-do list that would not take a significant amount of time but just hasn't happened yet. This year is all about making each day matter and living with the mindset that "procrastination is over and results are happening" so certainly don't rule out a goal that checks off the SMART boxes simply because it can be achieved quickly. It may help to think about it in terms of setting the three main goals as priorities you will look back on after BAR40 is complete and be able to have those as the top, bold headline of achievements.

I hope you'll find that using the SMART system as a type of litmus test to determine any weak spots or fault lines is a simple and effective step in confirming the sustainability of a goal as well as bringing to the surface any aspects of it that may derail it.

One final point of note on goal setting and a limitation of the SMART system: it is not GIGO proof. By that, I refer to the tried and true computer programming acronym for Garbage In, Garbage Out. If you simply pick a few random objectives to do over the next year, it's possible they will pass the SMART test (maybe just squeaking by in the "R" section), but it will be a disservice to yourself by limiting what milestones and achievements you tackle this year. It's fundamentally important to take the time to try and connect with your future self on what success really means to you.

Exercise

BAR40 and exercise go hand in hand. There is simply no getting around that fact, and my hope is that statement doesn't come as a surprise or revelation as in, "Wait, I'm going to have to work out during this?!" If that does happen to be your initial reaction, then hopefully, I can help reframe your perspective on living an active lifestyle and point out some facts that will chip away at the reluctance or negative connotations you have around working out.

On the other side of the coin, if exercise and fitness are already a part of your lifestyle, then this is a component of BAR40 that is really going to resonate as it will be a continuation and extension of what you are currently doing.

First off, whatever camp you may be in regarding exercise . . . love it, leave it, or somewhere in between let's do a quick refresher on some of the top reasons to exercise and why it's a game-changer in our lives on all levels.

In no particular order, here are some of the main benefits of exercise in broad terms:

- *Exercise will make you a happier person*
  Who doesn't want a natural boost of happiness, right? Both cardio and strength training have long been proven to boost mood. Research shows that within five minutes of starting cardio, your brain is releasing "feel-good" chemicals that include serotonin and dopamine. When

we work out, our bodies are also producing endorphins that interact with the brain and have effects that can be compared to morphine. Essentially, they help to dull workout-related pain and also deliver an overall sense of well-being. These euphoric feelings related to endorphins are widely thought to create the "runner's high" sensation you may have likely heard about or experienced first-hand. This general feeling of positivity and "all is well in the world" tends to stick around after the workout, so in that sense, it's the gift that keeps on giving. It's not hard to see how exercise is habit-forming in the sense that not only do we know it's the right thing to be doing from a health perspective, but it also makes us feel pretty great while we're doing it and as an added bonus we're going to have that great feeling stick around for a while after we're done. The good news here is that even if you don't have time for a full workout, even a five-minute walk is enough to trigger a quick mood boost.

- ***Working out decreases stress and anxiety levels***
  When it comes to writing about stress, it's one of those timeless topics. A statement like "in stressful times like these" would find a reader nodding in agreement in 1820 as sure as in 2020. Stress has always been a part of all our lives and comes in various forms. Stress is basically our body's reaction to any change that requires an adjustment or response, so it's easy to understand how we are dealing with some form of it on a continuous basis. Of course, not all stress is bad, and it serves a valuable purpose in heightening our situational awareness, keeping us

motivated, alert, and generally speaking, on top of our game. Consider events like a job interview or promotion, the birth of a child, or a whitewater rafting trip. All good things that our body will interpret as stressors and react to accordingly as the human brain has been hard-wired to do.

That said, often, when we think about the word "stress" the first thing that comes to mind is the negative connotation of the word and the emotions that go along with it. When one of our friends uses descriptions like: "stressed out," "high stress," "stressful," or "under stress" we know right away what they're talking about and can probably relate to those terms on a personal level having experienced times like that. We remember them because stress is often associated with being anxious or worried and, in general, not a pleasant feeling!

Through evolutionary improvements that span the ages, our body has become highly adept at dealing with a specific threat in the moment with a fight or flight response. That being the case, it may mean our reaction to someone honking the horn at us is probably still similar to the response we would have had back in the days of fighting off a rival hunter attempting to lay claim to a saber-toothed tiger we just successfully hunted.

What we are not well-suited for is long term (chronic) stress that tends to settle into our lives and puts our body on perpetual high alert status. This continuous state of tension brought on by prolonged stressful periods brings about a multitude of physical reactions that can have significant negative effects. Simply put, if the body never gets the signal that it can return to its normal state and constantly stays on red alert status, the effects can range from sleep disturbance, digestive issues, high blood pressure, heart disease, decreased immunity functions and all of the corresponding issues that can contribute to health problems.

This is where exercise comes in as such a critical and effective way proven to be a powerful frontline defense system. Not only does exercise reduce the amounts of natural stress hormones in the body, specifically adrenaline and cortisol, it also increases endorphins, which provide mood-elevating benefits. In addition, regular exercise leads to better sleep, which also goes a long way toward warding off the effects of stress. So speaking of sleep . . .

- ***Working out will help you sleep better***
Often neglected and frequently the first account we borrow from for an emergency time loan, the hugely important work that sleep does should give it the "unsung hero" designation in our daily lives. Some of the main benefits that come from sleep include increased concentration and mental functions, maximized physical performance, helping regulate body weight, strengthening the immune system, increased memory retention, and helping the body heal. I imagine sleep to be like a professional pit crew on a racetrack, and those hours of rest we get each night is when the team is out working on all the fixes and improvements. But if it's so great, why are we chronically short on it as a nation? I

think part of the problem is that while many things on our daily to-do list have a clear beginning and endpoint and can be easily categorized as "started, in-progress, or completed," that's not the case for sleep. Whether it's a workout, mowing the lawn, or bingeing a new season of something on Netflix . . . these activities all have a defined start and stop to them. With sleep, we tend to treat it as an afterthought and like to-do list table scraps; whatever time is left in our day we toss over and check off sleep as "done" on our list.

Speaking from personal experience, sleep was always the first thing to be sacrificed on any given day that I needed extra time to finish other tasks. Like most of us, I was certainly aware of the CDC suggested guidelines of seven-plus hours per night (adults 18-60) but dismissed it with the justification that I felt fine with 4-5 hours a night. Full disclosure, at one point years ago, I read an article about "short-sleeper" syndrome, which affects about 1-3 percent of the population and is characterized by minimal nightly sleep requirements to achieve "fully-rested" status. I was partially convinced that I fell into that category and felt fortunate to possibly be in that lucky minority bestowed with a productivity-boosting superpower. Long story short, that theory did not withstand much scrutiny. There are some fairly simple ways to check for yourself in the case you may be having similar thoughts (just Google "Super Sleeper" or "Short Sleeper" and you'll have plenty to read). The main self-test involves creating an optimal sleep environment free of possible light or sound interruptions and allowing yourself to sleep until your body naturally awakes.

How long you sleep in that sort of test scenario can show a lot. For example, it showed that I would easily sleep seven hours instead of the five I was used to getting, thereby indicating I was not a true "short sleeper," just someone actively practicing sleep deprivation. The good news is a test that requires only to sleep, if possible, with any potential interruptions removed is not an unpleasant concept. The bad news is that in most scenarios, especially when we have children in the house, the luxury of this test is not conducive to repetitive experimenting!

There does seem to be a widespread and long overdue movement toward devoting more attention to "sleep hygiene" and improving our sleep habits. This is a far cry from the old battle cries of "sleep is for the weak" or "I'll sleep when I'm dead" that went along with the idea that sleeping more than the absolute bare minimum was a character flaw and form of laziness.

Speaking for my own approach to improving my sleep schedule (which needed a long-overdue overhaul) I have made it one of my BAR40 goals for the year, which means I am actively prioritizing and tracking my progress regarding getting more sleep. I've found that the simple first step of committing to it as an area of improvement goes a long way in keeping it in the front of my thoughts at night with an eye on the clock and always doing the math of when I need to head to bed to try and get seven hours. (Of course, there are apps and reminder alarms readily available for that 30-minute bedtime countdown nudge.)

Another great tool I use is the Fitbit. Like many wearable fitness tracking devices, it has sleep monitoring capabilities which provide a summary report in the morning of all sorts of good stuff you missed while you were out. Top headlines include:

- Percentage of spent in sleep stages: awake, light, REM and deep
- Restoration: basically, how restful your sleep was based on tossing and turning, sleeping heart rate and estimated oxygen variation
- Graph display of interruptions in your sleep and at what points you woke up

Above all else, my go-to detail to check in the morning is my sleep score. This is a numeric value up to 100 with corresponding excellent, good, fair, and poor brackets. The overall score is a summary of the measured areas (sleep duration, depth, and restoration), and from a self-competition standpoint, it provides a perfect target to beat every day. If you already track your sleep, then you probably know what I mean when I say it's a great feeling to start off the day with a small victory of beating your sleep score from the day before.

The bottom line for me when it comes to sleep, with or without technology: it's a straightforward and worthwhile goal to be sure sleep is a top priority of your healthy living program. How well rested we are is a foundation that so many of our waking efforts are built upon, so it's an enormous advantage to be sure we take care of that fundamental need as it will continue to pay dividends.

It's safe to say and easy to agree that there are plenty of awesome reasons to exercise and plenty of benefits that go along with an active lifestyle. I suspect this isn't a revelation to you, but as mentioned at the top, I wanted to summarize some of the main elements that keep me motivated on a daily basis . . . especially on a day where working out is not at the top of your list of things you feel like doing.

On the topic of working out . . . the question you may have regarding BAR40 may be something along the lines of what do I need to do? So let's shed some light on that topic.

I think it helps to include some historical context of the original BAR40 plan. It gives insight that will hopefully provide some clarity on the importance of your main objective versus a "must do" approach. As mentioned at the start, I created BAR40 with the mentality that I wanted to use my 40th year to get into the best shape of my life. One of the obvious components of that was going to include losing some weight as I had packed on some gradual pounds over the years that I was not liking the look of. I wasn't exactly sure how much weight I needed to lose, but in keeping with the idea of SMART goals, I knew I needed a specific target weight. One thing I did was to look back at old photos and found a version of myself that looked like a weight I would like to get back to. As a longtime runner, I've always kept running journals that had my weekly weight included in them so once I found a photo that I liked with my slimmer self in it, I looked at the date stamp (May of 2000/age 24) and cross-referenced it to the corresponding year's running journal to determine what my actual weight was at the time. Lo and behold, "surprise" would be a major understatement when I dug that year's running journal out of an old storage box and found that my weight in the photo would have been 165. At that moment I was tipping the scales at 209 . . . somehow in the last 16 years, I had managed to add a mind-bending 44 lbs. Suffice to say, this was a disturbing revelation that brought on a mix of responses starting with what you may expect. First, some good old fashioned "well, that can't be right" denial. Once again, thanks to the tracked weight in my running journals, it didn't take much advanced detective work to flip around the months and see that yes, that was definitely the correct weight and in fact, I could watch it on the pages gradually going up in very small increments over the months and years. Looking back at the day it really was a slightly disturbing exercise with the major underlying question of "how on earth did this happen?" repeating in my mind. After the denial came the thought of "well, time to find a different picture" and lower my sights at what my target weight should be. This response automatically felt off and like a bit of surrender in the sense that I was essentially giving up on a goal simply because it seemed like it was going to be too much of a challenge, and of course, I did not want to set myself up for failure. Part of my brain was already looking for an escape hatch and was busy sending out Hail Mary attempts in the form of reminders about the SMART goal . . . It must be realistic! seemed like a subconscious shout. I was giving this a fair amount of thought in efforts to determine if it was, in fact, realistic because I really was committed to the idea of pursuing the "best year ever" and the idea of kicking it off with a modified weight goal that I watered-down to make more attainable was not sitting well with me. The one realization that pushed me to the "this is doable" side was thinking about my experience with Lent in previous years. I realized that any year I gave up drinking for Lent, I invariably dropped an average of 15 lbs. and that was only over the course of six weeks. Of course, it all came right back once Lent was over and I got back to my old beer-drinking ways, but as a concept, it made me wonder how much weight could be lost if I eliminated drinking for a whole year instead of just a month and a half. I also was having a candid look at what I was eating and realized my diet was an area that could also be significantly changed. Based on just the beer and food changes, I concluded the goal of 165 was, theoretically, realistic. Not an easy one, but possible, was my thinking. So with that, the decision was made.

In looking at the running journals, I could also see a distinct correlation between a decrease in my weekly mileage and my increase in weight over the years, especially noticeable from '09-'12. Our daughter was born in 2009, and as is often the case for new parents, the exercise time can take a hit on the schedule when there is a newborn around bringing all those new demands babies are so well known for. That part is understandable for a window of time, but what I was having a hard time reconciling is why my mileage did not return to normal weekly levels long after it could and should have. Habit is, of course, the answer. Over time, I simply got into the habit of running less every week. My metabolism apparently was okay in regulating my weight based on whatever I was eating and drinking when I was regularly running, but once I slashed my weekly caloric output, the engine slowed down, and the weight added up. No major revelations there, but the answer for me was crystal clear . . . I needed to start logging some more mileage again and do an overhaul on what fuel I was putting into my body.

So began what would be the framework for my BAR40 exercise plan. I was going to commit to a goal of 1500 miles for the year, with a weekly goal of 30 miles divided over five days. The actual mileage on any day could vary if, at the end of the week, the total hit 30. This approach checked off a couple of boxes for me. First, I had a SMART goal for the year in terms of mileage that was significantly more than the annual mileage of 1000-1200 that I had been averaging. Second, I had weekly goals in terms of how much mileage I needed to get in as well as breaking it down further to a minimum of five days running. My running log has always had the Monday-Sunday format, so if for some reason I wanted to take off Monday and Tuesday, then I knew I would be running the next five days. Or, if I wanted to run a shorter distance all seven days that week it worked too if I hit the 30 miles.

In addition, my personal fitness goal of getting in the best shape ever was more than just the number on the scale each week. I wanted to incorporate more of a full-body workout into my weekly routine as opposed to "leg day, every day" and add some muscle and definition without necessarily looking to bulk up.

This is an area where I was especially determined to come up with an effective plan. I knew what didn't work from previous experience and had clear ideas on how to fix the weak spots prone to failure. It's worth repeating here that BAR40 is based on creating habits that result in incremental improvements compounding over time. What we're shooting for is getting better in every way, every day. Having a process and routine that is sustainable over time is critical, and it's worth the effort to identify early on any obstacles that are blocking the way. Spotting and eliminating the potential threat to your routine is much more effective in the planning stage as opposed to once you are starting to get the momentum going and realize you need to rethink the plan and change things up.

For me, working out in the past involved using weights or gym equipment either in my basement or at an actual gym. As a concept, there's obviously nothing wrong with either of those scenarios, but I was finding that most times I was traveling for work, I would end up skipping any workout except for running. As I traveled for work frequently, this was something I knew would be an ongoing stumbling block to my goal of consistency. What about hotel gyms, you ask? They were always in the back of mind as an option, but in actuality, it was a rare occurrence for me to actually use one. Too small, too crowded, not open when I arrived at check-in . . . there are a bunch of excuses why I didn't use them, but the main takeaway is "know thyself" and the bottom line was I wasn't using them or likely to use them consistently. Having the self-awareness to spot the possible weak link in your fitness plan and addressing it in the interest of creating a goal is a major step in the right direction with regard to building a sustainable plan. Keep in mind, ideally you come up with an exercise schedule that you not only stick with but are also motivated to do for the next 52 weeks!

So in my case, I had the running part of my plan worked out as far as the weekly mileage goal and the way I would achieve it, but the gym workout was still a question mark. After looking at it from different angles and considering various less than perfect ideas (for instance, double workouts at home to make up for what I missed on the road . . . yikes) it occurred to me that my desire and commitment to work out were consistent, but the variable causing the inconsistency was an external factor . . . the gym. With that lightbulb moment came the clear realization that in order to make BAR40 a truly self-sustaining program, it should be designed to be completely independent of outside needs that could derail it. At the time, I was already doing some occasional push-ups, nothing consistent but enough to get me thinking in terms of how ideal they were as an exercise that could be done anywhere. That's what got me thinking about the concept of building an entire workout around bodyweight exercises as an alternative to the gym. Once I started looking into that, I was blown away at the number of options that were available.

Bear in mind, this was all going on in 2016. In the years since then there has been an explosion of fitness apps and streaming options on Netflix, YouTube, and Amazon Prime (to name just a few) that provide a whole galaxy of gym alternatives to be viewed, tracked and shared from the palm of your hand. Now added to the mix is the fact that gyms are/were temporarily closed during the Covid-19 crisis, which prompted a huge wave of new online content with ideas on how to keep active at home. When it comes to anything related to health and fitness, I'm all in—so I think it's awesome to see the steadily growing trend of people of all ages becoming more active. The idea of a healthy lifestyle is steadily becoming much more of a mainstream pursuit as we have all seen. Just look around to see how athleisure wear has become the default casual style. If you take a second to think about it, it wasn't really that long ago that if you were in workout gear while out running errands on a Saturday afternoon, you looked like someone who probably didn't go home to take a shower after the gym. Now, no one would give you a second look walking around Target in yoga tights or running pants. Also, pretty much gone from the 2020 vocabulary . . . the term "health nut." Remember that one?

At any rate, while the proliferation of home fitness options is awesome on a lot of levels, I go back to my original point on the importance of creating a workout plan that is not overly reliant on external factors. Or, if you do decide to design your BAR40 workout plan around a streaming service or fitness app, have a backup plan for those times where there's no Wi-Fi, your phone is dead, the internet is down or any other technology glitch that would disrupt your workout.

To get back to my initial point about the bodyweight exercise research I was doing in 2016, I found *You Are Your Own Gym* by Mark Lauren and the search was over.

First off, let me clarify that in no way am I any sort of paid spokesman for the book. I do not know Mark, have never spoken with him, and have no motive in endorsing his techniques and book other than the fact that I have personally used them and found that if you put the work in, you will without question see significant results. Overall, it's a fantastic resource.

Mark's background is as a trainer to the US Special Operations community, and his techniques are used by the Navy SEALs, Army Green Berets, and Air Force Special Tactics Operators and are a core component of their strength training programs. Some specific elements of Mark's training and resume make this fitness program especially well-suited for the BAR40 52-week duration. Shortly after 9/11 (the following week) Mark left his team (the 22nd Special Tactics Squadron) to become a full-time Military Physical Training Specialist. One of the realities of that time was a surge in demand for SpecOps soldiers that needed to be trained and deployed in a short period of time. The traditional physical training programs being used were effective but were not well-suited for the immediacy of requirements following 9/11. Mark helped revamp the program using the most modern sports-science principles and applied them to strength training and conditioning to deliver optimal results in the least amount of time. These programs also needed to include the latest thinking on recovery and progression to minimize the attrition rate, which ended up being reduced by 40% compared to the old training program. Every six weeks marked the arrival of a new incoming class of recruits that needed a short window of time to reach the required SpecOps physical training standards before deployment. The same techniques used in that training are made available in his book and are designed for one thing: to get you in the best shape possible. Another major point that shouldn't be overlooked is the fact that once you do achieve these results through these exercises for 52 weeks, the habits are going to be developed, and the exercises will be so familiar that it becomes a lifestyle. It's a huge benefit to have a full arsenal of bodyweight exercises at your disposal that can be done anywhere. You will, very literally, be able to get a full-body intense workout wherever you are at any time that works for you . . . no equipment or technology required.

In addition to Mark's history and proven success, here are some of the main benefits of making this book your go-to resource for strength training:

- 125 exercises designed to work for every fitness level from first time ever working out to competitive bodybuilder and the whole range in between

- The workouts can be done anywhere and are not subject to any external factor that can get in the way. Whether it's your bedroom, basement, garage, backyard, or hotel room you can be confident that you will get a full workout in without needing a trip to the gym or relying on the fitness equipment

- Pre-designed 10-week programs that are broken into four classes of advancing intensity: Basic (beginner), 1st Class (intermediate) Master (advanced) and Chief (elite). Each 10-week program is made up of four "blocks." Muscular Endurance is weeks 1 and 2; this uses "ladders" of low intensity but a higher amount of reps. Next is the Strength Training Block (weeks 3-4), which is higher intensity but fewer reps. Following that is Power Blocks (weeks 5-6), made up of the highest intensity and fewest reps. The last one is Undulating Block (weeks 7-10) which is a combination of all the earlier methods as well as some new ones.

- These programs are designed to deliver maximum results with military efficiency. All the blocks are based around 20- to 30-minute workouts 4-5 days a week (Blocks 1-3 are 4-day workouts and Block 4 is a 5-day plan). I've pointed out the main reason why I rely on bodyweight exercises as the central component of the BAR40 program, which is eliminating any obstacle to being able to get my workout done no matter where I am. It's amazing when you think about the fact that we have this amazing machine, the human body, that can reach its peak potential using all the tools that we already have. It's quite easy to get caught up in the nonstop barrage of marketing messages that we are constantly hit with for new pieces of equipment and fad programs that make wild promises for amazing results with virtually no effort. Fitness is big business, and the companies that make equipment have teams of talented people coming up with extremely effective campaigns designed to get us to buy that equipment . . . and no question about it, they're great at their job! Hence the reason why so many basements, garages and yard sales are littered with barely used gadgets and pieces of fitness equipment that did not come close to delivering results that looked anything like the commercial. It's also certainly true that a significant component of that failure in results is simply because often people buy these things with the intention of using them and for various reasons that doesn't happen.

The bottom line is most people have not spent time and energy in the training and dedication required to learn how to become skilled at using your own body to surpass the results that you're looking for elsewhere. Power, speed, endurance, balance, flexibility, cardiovascular health, strength . . . these are all things the human body is designed for! It's easy to lose sight of the fact that since humans have been walking the earth, our standard equipment gives us all the tools we need to be at peak performance. In the grand scheme of time, it's a relatively recent development where we have become a much more sedentary species that relies less on our bodies and more on our minds. Obviously, the days of humans evading natural predators in the wild while hunting for food are long gone, but in much more recent times, exercise and activity levels have trended downward while eating habits have taken a turn for the worse with food quality and larger portions. While that may be the 2021 reality we live in, it doesn't mean that we have to simply be a passenger along for the ride. More than ever, it means we need to be diligent in having a plan in place that ensures we take care of ourselves and adopt the mindset that we have all the tools we need available to us 24/7 to reach and maintain the best physical version of ourselves.

All that said, it's obvious that I'm an advocate of incorporating bodyweight exercises into your exercise plan for the next year, but of course, this is your BAR40 and only you should decide how you want to manage it with the "know thyself" filter on. Most importantly is giving thought to how you want to structure and plan your exercise program in a way that is going to motivate you and be effective in delivering results. Like everything else in BAR40, the exercise component is a self-guided journey with the ultimate intent of delivering results that will be considered *your* best year ever. This once again comes back to creating a SMART goal around your fitness ideals and should include activities that work for you and of course, what you want to achieve (weight loss, muscle definition, more stamina, first 5k . . . first marathon, etc.). Whether it's walking, biking, running, yoga, swimming, hiking, rollerblading (and yes, of course, the gym, if that's your thing!), the concept of fitness during BAR40 is that you take it to the next level. Frequency, intensity, duration, and consistency are the main areas I suggest you look at and build your plan around that.

Last but not least, on the subject of bodyweight exercises: a common misconception is that they only work certain muscle groups or are limited in difficulty. First, I would say that this book contains 125 exercises, which leaves no muscle left behind. Secondly, variations can be applied to the exercises to provide a range of difficulty levels. Take an example like the push-up. (For the record, this underrated exercise works the chest, shoulders, triceps, abs, obliques, and lower back.) An entry-level version would be standing facing a wall; pretty basic stuff for someone starting out. After that, there is no shortage of variations that go way up on the difficulty scale. For example, before you dismiss the push-up as not tough enough to count as working out, try one-handed floor push-ups with your hand on an unstable surface (a basketball, for instance) and your feet on the couch. Repeat as necessary!

Consistency is such a critical component to building the habits that will help you achieve success in this area. As a related side note and using push-ups as a current example . . . an easy option for quick daily "bonus reps" is using your phone alarm set at times throughout the day. I have mine set to go off on the hour every hour 12 hours a day. When it goes off, it's a reminder to do 25 push-ups. It's not a lot obviously, but it's a super quick way to get a micro-workout in hourly and adds an additional 300 push-ups to my day in addition to whatever workout/run I'm doing (the 300 is based on doing 10 of the 12 hours which builds accounts for a couple times during that day when I can't do them or just don't want to). Some days I mix it up and do 50 every other hour and/or add in crunches to the push-ups; either way, the whole thing only takes about a minute. As a great example of habit, start doing that hourly alarm and you'll be amazed how fast push-ups become part of your routine throughout the day. Don't worry about getting some in around your friends; you may be surprised how many will join you. Back to the topic of consistency . . . as you have almost certainly heard and possibly experienced, New Year's resolutions around exercise are overwhelmingly failed attempts with statistics showing that 80% are abandoned efforts by the second week of February. In 2019 Strava did some research of its own using data from millions of user-logged activities and came up with January 19th as the date that most people give up on their resolution. They even came up with a name for it: Quitters Day. These statistics come as no surprise. Most of these plans are made with good intentions but are doomed for failure before they ever begin. As the saying goes, a goal without a plan is just a wish, and I would argue that most resolutions have not even passed the SMART process to qualify them as viable goals. Most importantly, though, the failure to launch is more around the power of habits and the fact that these failed attempts do not factor in building the habit around it.

Let's make no mistake about it: committing to 52 weeks of increased working out is not an easy feat. BAR40 is meant to be challenging, and I know with certainty that the person you are at the end of it will be You 2.0 on a lot of levels, but the critical first step is laying the foundation for the habits that will help ensure you steer far clear of that 80% statistic of people who throw in the towel. This is the main reason that I have *The Power of Habit* as the first book on the BAR40 reading list. It provides amazing insights on how the brain works with regard to the "habit loop" (cue, routine, reward) of creating or breaking cycles in our daily life. More on that later, but most importantly, the book will provide beneficial insights toward ensuring your fitness goals will be achieved. Creating the habit of personal accountability to your future self where failure is not an option and that you are going to stick with this no matter what is so important . . . do not give yourself an escape hatch! That mentality, along with using habit-building tools will get you well on the way, and once momentum is on your side and the fitness routine habit has taken hold, it becomes infinitely easier and simply part of your weekly routine.

To summarize the whole topic of exercise, the bottom line is to identify what activities you currently enjoy or would like to begin and create a weekly schedule that will guarantee that they happen. Building a habit of personal accountability in making sure you are achieving your weekly fitness objective is critical to the success of using this year to reach your optimal fitness level. Your daily and weekly exercise need to become a protected priority that is a non-negotiable commitment to yourself.

As I mentioned about sleep, it's often too easy to put working out in the front of the line of daily activities that are sacrificed or cut short in order to meet some other need that pops up. It goes without saying—there will be times when something unexpected happens that requires you to miss a planned workout, and I'm not referring to those situations. My point is that in order to get the results you are looking for, consistency is key, especially when the habit is forming. Choosing what exercise(s) you are going to do each week (running, biking, walking, swimming, etc.) and building a schedule that realistically fits into your life is the main step. Only you know your current physical fitness baseline and limitations, so use that (or check with your doctor if unsure) to determine your frequency, duration, and intensity. If you can manage to set a 4- or 5-day-a-week schedule that includes a workout, that would be a challenging goal that will take you to the next level. If you are currently working out with that level of frequency, then the objective will be incrementally adding to the duration, distance, and intensity of the workouts to reach new milestones. Bear in mind that from an injury avoidance perspective, there needs to be a progression of increase and not an overnight or rapid change. For instance, a rule of thumb with running is adding no more than 10% mileage increases per week. You can easily find recommended increase guidelines for whatever your activity of choice is. Whatever activity you are doing or plan on doing, the objective is to do more of it on a weekly basis over the duration of BAR40 than you have ever done before . . . safely and for the long haul! It does us no good to ramp up our workout to the point of developing an overuse injury that will sideline the entire effort.

If it helps you at all with examples of exercise goals, below is the fitness overview of my first year doing BAR40. I continued with running as one of my main activities but put some specific goals around it with regard to how many days I was going to run (5) and what the weekly miles were going to be (30) while factoring in the annual target. My target goal was 1500 miles, and I ended up reaching 1650 based on the fact that I ended up with higher mileage weeks when I was doing double runs to avoid peak heat in the summer.

I also added the bodyweight exercise component to my exercise regimen with a minimum goal of 20 days per month, which I would track in my journal. (When I was first starting these exercises and prone to making excuses to procrastinate or skip them, I would use a technique from *The Power of Habit* book on creating an unavoidable trigger. For this, I would put my workout mat on the floor next to my bed and would not allow myself to get into bed that night until the workout was done . . . simple but effective, and after a couple months that habit was fully formed, and the mat trick was no longer needed.)

I also wanted to be able to do 10 pull-ups. Starting out, I could barely do one without some air kicking and flailing, so to me, that was a big goal. (For those of you who can do 10 pull-ups without breaking a sweat and are shaking your head at what you consider an insignificant upper body strength goal, I point out that I'm sharing these to show that no fitness goal is wrong as long as it's important to you on the way to your best self . . . no judgment zone!) To help build the habit and repetition I put a basic, pressure mounted doorway pull-up bar in a high traffic area of my house as a constant reminder and used it throughout the day, every day, and like everything else pull-ups became easier over time until I could do 10.

In wrapping up this section, my starting weight was 209, and I had a target goal of 165. Through the combination of changing my diet (more on that soon) and putting this exercise program in place (running and bodyweight exercises), at week 52 I weighed in at 161 for a total loss of 48 lbs. In addition to the weight loss, the bodyweight exercises did exactly what they were supposed to do to create the more lean, muscular, and fit version of myself that I was shooting for.

Last, but definitely not least, was the unexpected overhaul on my health numbers. Based on my before and after blood panels that come with my annual physical, my blood pressure went from 125/80 to 105/65, my resting heart slowed from about 75 to 60, and my cholesterol dropped from 205 to 170. Without question or hesitation, I can say that at the end of my 40th year, I was in the best shape of my life, and I'm still amazed at the power of the BAR40 program in reaching that outcome.

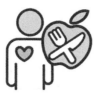

Diet

As I write this in late November 2020, our world is one of change and uncertainty in many areas including Covid-19, climate, politics, and the economy just to rattle off a shortlist . . . but one constant we have now and have had for thousands of years—literally, thousands of years—is the topic of diet. Over 2,400 years ago, Hippocrates, the OG of medicine, wrote, "Man cannot live healthily on food, they need a certain amount of exercise." His instruction to obese patients was to exercise until exhaustion and then eat while out of breath. Tough love!

Around the world, weight loss is a topic that has always had plenty of interested followers and, lacking evidence to suggest otherwise, always will. Despite thousands of years of advice, concepts, approaches, fads, and gimmicks, there is a constant influx of new "target audience" members. Here in the US that audience is growing in more ways than one. According to the CDC, the percentage of Americans that are now categorized as obese has reached 42.4% (based on their latest survey in 2018) which is up from 30.5% in 2000. (In the 1960's, the percentage was less than 20% so as a nation Americans became really big, really quick). Also steadily on the rise is the valuation of the US weight loss industry, which hit $72 billion in 2019, showing 4% growth over 2018. You would think that any problem that had so many billions of dollars spent on fixing it would, at a minimum, show signs of improvement instead of gradually worsening, but that is not the case with losing weight. Malcolm Gladwell wrote an interesting and well-publicized article about this trend way back in 1998 called "The Pima Paradox" in which he pointed out that although loads of new diet books were cranked out each year, there was a repeating formula that many of the authors followed. Gladwell calls it a "540-degree rhetorical triple-gainer," since it involves making six claims:

- It's a myth you must suffer
- Yes, all the books say that
- Of course, you don't believe them
- I was like you, convinced I had to suffer to lose weight
- Because it's true
- Unless you use my diet, which involves no suffering at all

While I'm not an avid reader of diet books, I have no doubt that Gladwell's findings are spot on as it seems to make sense in the context that we live in a society that puts a high premium on instant gratification regardless of the pursuit. Results without effort are more often than not an aspiration doomed to failure, and ample evidence is provided by the statistics around "fad diets" (defined by Wikipedia as: "a diet popular for a time without being a standard dietary recommendation, and often promising unreasonably fast weight loss or nonsensical health improvements").

BAR40 is by no means a diet book, and I have no interest in joining the incredibly overcrowded market of publications already out there. While there are surely plenty of great plans that help people get the results they're looking for, it's also safe to say that there is also a long list that make wild promises backed up by pseudo-science and questionable research. If losing weight is your main goal in doing BAR40, then hopefully I will succeed in helping cut through the clutter of what I imagine to be a frustrating gauntlet of different and contra-dictory options: Paleo, Atkins, Whole30, fasting, keto-genic, DASH, Mediterranean, MIND, juicing, low-FODMAP, GOLO Diet, 1200 calorie diet, Dubrow Diet, Sebi Diet, Sirtfood Diet, Endomorph Diet . . . you get the idea. It's really a head-spinning list, and that's just looking at 2019 diet trends! It's no wonder that so many people pinball back and forth trying to find a plan that works for them and, statistically speaking, consis-tently fail to achieve the results they're looking for. My goal here is only to share what my approach is and provide some resources that proved to be highly effective for me when I decided to get back to my target weight and lose a considerable number of pounds. Even more importantly, I have a solid belief that with the commitment of adopting a revised approach to your diet, these will become habits that will help ensure you maintain your target weight and avoid the eventual return of the weight that on average happens to the slow tune of a few pounds per year.

So to get back to Gladwell's point about the "no suffering" claims that are so commonly tossed around in diet books, I want to be clear that while I wouldn't go so far as to call it "suffering" (we are talking about food here, not a chainsaw accident) some changes definitely need to happen in order to get to where you want to end up. Sacrifices will be made, and it's a perfect chance to get more comfortable being uncomfortable, but at the same time, the plan needs to be sustainable for the long haul, many years after BAR40 is done.

Much like the earlier example about having your workout be dependent on using a gym, when there are additional outside requirements needed for your diet plan to be effective, it adds to the risk of possible factors that can send the plan off track. What I consider the greatest strength of the approach of BAR40 is that it is based on extremely straightforward concepts that are universally applied across each meal and snack regardless of your dietary preferences (vegan, dairy free, gluten free, etc.). Basically, it's a very simple concept, but not always mentally easy.

Mainly, the approach is based on substitution, reduction of your sugar intake, and calibrating the "full" mark on your fuel tank. That's it, there really isn't much more to the approach, and the beauty of it is that once the substitutions are made, your tastes will adapt to the new normal. This diminishes the constant cravings that some may refer to as the suffering part. The whole concept is that all these small changes add up to significant differences over time, which will ultimately make that healthy substitution an automatic function, as is the case with other habits.

Really, what we are ultimately building and reinforcing is a mindset much more than any "diet plan" in the traditional sense of the term. This approach—looking at what we are eating through the lens of, how can I change this to be better—creates an amazing snowball effect that continues to build momentum over time. Each small change brings an incremental benefit, and the next small change and benefit build on the one before it, making the combined benefits slightly greater.

Think of it like compound interest, which Albert Einstein has described as the eighth wonder of the world, summarizing it by saying, "He who understands it, earns it... he who doesn't, pays it." Warren Buffet, who is widely considered to be one of the most successful investors of all time, sums it up with, "My wealth has come from a combination of living in America, some lucky genes and compound interest."

The same concept that applies to financial growth—interest on top of interest builds wealth at an accelerated rate—applies to life, which of course includes healthy choices in our diet. All the small positive changes accumulate to the extent that while you have done a significant overhaul on your daily diet, it doesn't feel like you are torturing yourself because in general you are still eating what you want . . . just better versions.

Let's start with a main offender in the average American diet: added sugars. There are many areas we as Americans can proudly say that we are #1 in and this is not one of them. To be clear, we are #1 . . . the world leader in sugar consumption, but it's definitely not anything to brag about. It's no coincidence that the US also holds the #1 spot in obesity levels. Our sugar intake and obesity statistics have steadily tracked upward together over the years, and we are now very much living in the land of the sugar addicted. There is no getting around the fact . . . sugar is tough to avoid unless we are making a conscious effort to do so. It is, quite literally, in virtually everything we buy at the grocery store with three out of four items on the shelf or in the cooler containing some form of added sugar.

Here are some statistics from the Diabetes Council:

- There are 4.2 grams of sugar in a teaspoon, and the average daily US consumption per person is around 126 grams, or 30 teaspoons. Recommended US daily dietary guidelines limit added sugar to 10%, not exceeding 12 teaspoons. 90% of Americans consume more than the daily recommended amount of sugar.

- Sugar is related to all sorts of medical problems, but some of the main ones are obesity, hypertension, heart and liver diseases, Type 2 diabetes, and not to be forgotten, tooth decay.

- A 10-year study ending in 2018 published in the Atlantic shows that people with high blood sugar levels have a much faster cognitive decline than those with normal blood sugar. Those with Type 2 Diabetes at the beginning of the study were twice as likely to develop Alzheimer's.

While sugar may be all around us, our main source of it comes in liquid form. By far, sugary drinks have become the primary delivery system for the majority of Americans' daily dose. For the age bracket of 12-50, drinks represent 46% of daily sugar intake with snacks and sweets in second place at 31%.

Harvard School of Public Health published some interesting findings on sugary drinks, and it refers to the trend as "supersizing and the obesity epidemic." Essentially, over the years, our drink sizes have gotten enormous. Before the 1950's drink sizes were 6.5 ounces; in the 50's the 12-ounce size was introduced, in the 90's the 20-ounce bottle became prominent, and in the present day, it is not uncommon to see fountain drinks and travel mugs in the one-liter size. As you likely already know, the vast majority of these drinks that keep getting bigger are sugar drinks, so the bigger the bottle, the more teaspoons of sugar we get every day. Soda (or "pop" depending on where you live) tends to emerge as the main villain in any study on sugary drinks, and it deserves the spotlight based on how large a role it plays as our American beverage of choice.

Not to be overlooked, though, are all the other drinks ending with 'ade, including sports drinks that are loaded with sugar. As a diet modification starting point, I would highly recommend taking a hard look at what you are drinking every day and how you can improve it by reducing the amount of sugar . . . and that includes all of its many forms and variations including anything that ends with 'ose on the ingredient list (dextrose, sucrose, high-fructose corn syrup, maltose, etc.)!

Obviously, the best bet is water—we all know that—but the problem is from a taste perspective, water isn't a psychologically acceptable substitute. Going from super sweet water to boring, flat water is a big leap. One option is adding some fruit slices to the water to punch it up with your favorite flavor. (Wait, you shout, . . . fruit has sugars! That's a reasonable point, and to that, I would say the goal here is not to eliminate all sugar consumption; it's to drastically reduce added sugars. Natural sugars occurring in a healthy diet come along with vitamins and minerals too, unlike the added sugars which have no nutritional value.)

Another option, and definitely my go-to drink of choice day and night, is seltzer. Cold, crisp, bubbling, and refreshing seltzer naturally flavored in choices to satisfy virtually every taste. It really is a fantastic option that can be the go-to substitute for whatever you're drinking. All the taste and fizz of soda with 0 calories, 0 sweeteners, 0 sugars. That said, I recognize that sugar is an addictive substance, and someone with an established daily soda habit may have a tough time kicking it cold turkey. For example, I have a close friend (we'll call him Art) who is a super-bright guy, avid biker, skier, and runner with an overall very healthy lifestyle. Also, as an ER doctor, he sees obesity-related medical maladies first-hand on a regular basis and knows the havoc too much sugar can bring. All that said, Art has a love of soda—Mountain Dew in particular, a devilish concoction even by the low and loose standards of the soda industry. Art has struggled over the years to kick that habit and has mostly gotten there through substitution efforts.

If you can do the hard stop on the sugar drinks and switch to an alternative like seltzer, awesome . . . that's a major and immediate diet improvement! If you want to transition over, set up a reduction plan where you're doing a ratio of your drink of choice with added seltzer or water. If you do a 50/50 split to start off with, then no matter what, at the end of each week you just reduced by half the amount of sugar you drank. That plan could be on a reducing schedule so that within a few weeks you're doing a 75/25 ratio and ultimately eliminating it altogether.

As far as all the other sugars in your diet are concerned, once you start being mindful of trying to reduce it, you can find ways to limit your intake all around. Coffee is another easy target. Think about that one . . . do you really need to be ordering coffee with added sugar? In so many cases our taste buds have grown very accustomed to the super high level of sweetness that is found across the board in so many foods and drinks, but I tell you with absolute surety that given the chance your tastes will adjust to the new normal without all the excess sweetener taste. Using coffee as an example, I grew up in Massachusetts, where Dunkin' is king, and the standard order includes cream and sugar. When I switched from that blend to skim milk with no sugar, it was definitely a huge flavor difference (no question, it was not a particularly good one on first sip). Since I drank a lot of coffee, I gave my palate plenty of opportunities to get acclimated to the reality and within a few weeks I did not give it a second thought. My taste buds had forgotten all about the old coffee version. Fast forward to now, if I order a coffee and someone inadvertently made it with sugar, it tastes so sweet that it's not even something I would want to drink. Your tastes will change, and what originally seemed like a sacrifice on the taste side will become what you actually enjoy. Stick with it, and you will see what I mean.

While beverages may represent where we get most of our excess daily sugar every day, no doubt about it, food has plenty to spare as well. The simple answer is—and this is the part where some radical change is often required—take a hard look at what you're snacking on throughout the day and eliminate or replace it.

This gets back to my earlier point and my main approach at looking at what our normal diet is and making it better. This is something you can start immediately, meal by meal and snack by snack . . . grab a pad and pen and on one side, write out the foods you normally have, on the other side come up with a couple ideas for improving it and/or reducing it. This is your diet, so it has to be something you are on-board with in order for it to work on a daily basis. There is plenty of data that concludes diet plans that look great on paper but do not appeal to you have a well-established failure rate. Eating only grapefruit, celery sticks and croutons for a month would probably cause you to drop some pounds, but in most cases, it wouldn't be a realistic lifestyle diet that would stand the test of time. Again, small changes and modifications will add up and be sustainable for the long haul. The goal is not some miracle plan that would be tough to do for a week, let alone a year. Don't set yourself up for failure with some wildly unrealistic goals . . . eat what you like to eat but change it up so it's less fat, calories, and sugar and weight loss results will happen, and you will feel better overall in the process.

When you're shopping for ingredients at home, look for the low-fat options and look at what flavor substitutions can be used to lower the fat and sugar components. For ideas on recipes, try using applesauce instead of sugar, cut back on the amount of oils, use skim instead of whole milk. Instead of always using store-bought condiments and dressings, look at making some of them yourself. You control the ingredients, and it's pretty cool to find easy alternatives you can whip up at home with little effort, and that will probably save you money in the long run.

If it helps at all, below are some personal examples from my own diet that work for me and have been food habits for years at this point. (Or, if you really don't care what I eat, feel free to skip ahead . . . no offense taken!)

Breakfast

Old options: Bagels/cream cheese, omelets, home fries, "fruit on the bottom" yogurt, waffles with butter/syrup, orange juice. *Replaced with:* English muffin with low-fat cream cheese or natural peanut butter (thin layers, no need for a ½ inch base!), egg white omelet (no cheese), non-fat Greek yogurt with some added strawberries or blueberries and granola (keep an eye on the granola ingredients though, as a lot of store stuff is basically a sugar cereal packaged as granola, or bake your own). I got away from the waffles for the most part, but when I do, I skip the butter and use a small amount of syrup, none of that "Lake Maple" pouring approach. Also, instead of butters, I use Brummel & Brown, a butter substitute.

Lunch

Old options: I would usually go for some sort of sandwich or fast food meal. Lunch can be a tough one if you're at work and going out to grab something from a local place, but it's certainly manageable.

Replaced with: I usually have a protein bar for lunch, although this is another food category that warrants some attention to ingredients. Over the years, this has become an area with an abundance of options, and a lot of them are basically candy bars packaged to look like a healthy alternative. I tend to go with Think bars as they taste good, have a short ingredient list, are high on protein and low on sugar. If I'm going out to lunch somewhere, I'll get a turkey sandwich or grilled chicken, no cheese or mayo . . . just some lettuce, tomato, or mustard. If I want some chips, I'll get something liked Baked Lays or the best available option. I'm not big on salads, but if that's your thing, getting the dressing on the side is an easy way to manage that added element that packs a big punch with fat and sugar content.

Dinner

When it comes to restaurants, this is the meal when most of us probably end up going out to eat, which is always a challenge with regard to keeping your good intentions on track. I don't have an old versus new list here except for the approach that I try to make whatever I'm ordering as healthy as possible. Skipping the cheese is always an easy option, getting something in a wrap instead of a bun usually works, swapping fries for a salad, getting the baked potato condiments on the side instead of pre-loaded, avoiding fried appetizers, keeping the breadbasket visits to a minimum . . . all small changes that through repetition will become an extremely easy change that will not leave you "suffering" (to use that old word) and delivers results that add up in big ways . . . especially if you frequently enjoy restaurants.

One big change you can make is also a simple one . . . take some of it home. A general trend that you have likely noticed is portion sizes at restaurants have grown over the years. While you can look at that as a positive development from a dollar value perspective, it often means we end up eating way more than we should. Let's face it: our natural inclination is to finish the food that's put in front of us . . . it seems to be a hardwired response most of us have and probably comes from that message repeatedly being drilled into us at our childhood dinner tables. This is a great area to think about and work on as we often have the habit of eating until we feel physically full, which, especially if we eat fast, is way more than we actually need at any given meal. On some level, our brain is still wired for survival mode in that when we encounter food, we need to consume as much as possible in the event that it's a long time before we are able to successfully hunt and kill another saber-toothed tiger and ward off starvation.

For most of us reading this, the availability of our next meal is not something in question, but we still tend to eat as if it may be a while before we have another chance. If you can get into the habit of taking some of the meal home with you, the benefits are easy to see. You end up having a much more appropriate sized portion; you don't leave feeling stuffed; you'll feel that small feeling of victory knowing you did the right (if not easy) thing; and you'll end up getting two meals for your money instead of one. If it helps, when you're ordering, just ask the server to pack up half the meal to go; that way, when your dinner comes out, you can still finish what's on your plate without thinking about it. This can be a good approach if you're out with a group of friends, so you don't have to stare at half a plate of food (or keep picking at it) while everyone else is eating. It also eliminates any of the "not hungry?" or "what, no good?" questions that may come up. Never having the food on the plate in the first place helps avoid those annoying conversations. Another tip on the restaurant topic is having a small healthy snack at home before you head out to dinner. This is based on the fact that when you show up at the restaurant famished, you're that much more likely to eat more bread and appetizers while you're waiting for the entree to come out. From the time you leave your house, get your table at the restaurant, order, and your meal is actually placed in front of you, a couple of hours can go by, so pre-planning that window of time instead of leaving the house ravenous is a worthwhile strategy.

As far as dinner at home, for anything that requires ground meat, I use 99% fat-free ground turkey or chicken. If we're making burgers, we'll go with lean ground beef. I tend to have one meal more than any other, which is turkey Manwich (aka sloppy joe) sandwiches. I happen to think they taste great (obviously, which is why it's my go-to meal), but they're also easy to cook and a great healthy option. If you're looking to try them, the shopping list is simple: 1 pound 99% fat free turkey, 1 packet McCormick Sloppy Joe seasoning, 1 6-ounce can of tomato paste (I use Hunt's No Salt Added). I usually have it on toasted rye bread with pickles (dill "stackers") and some horseradish. If you want some fries with it, my preferred choice is Nathan's, which has a relatively low fat content when it comes to frozen fry choices. I use an air fryer, and they come out as crispy and golden brown as if you just got them on the boardwalk at Coney Island! Another option on the fries is to simply cut up a regular baking potato in fry size slices, put them in a zip lock bag with a little bit of oil and seasoning of your choice (salt and pepper or Old Bay are good), shake them up and bake for 20 minutes in the air fryer if you have one (or just the regular oven works fine, too). If you're like me and are perfectly happy with the same meal multiple times in the week, another good option is to use a rice cooker to make a good size batch of rice and also steam some broccoli or veggie of your choice. Grill up enough chicken breasts for however many portions you want to make, and you will have enough grilled chicken, steamed rice, and veggies to last you for multiple meals.

Last but not least: dessert. If I had a favorite, it would probably be ice cream, so my go-to option with that is fat free, no sugar vanilla frozen yogurt. You may think . . . boring! But again, it all comes down to how your tastes adjust over time. To me, that tastes great and does not seem like I'm sacrificing anything (go crazy and add some strawberries or blueberries!). If you're into cookies, bake some using a healthy recipe for a better alternative. The sugar-free cookie recipes that are easily found online are delicious alternatives to the store-bought stuff and a breeze to make. My point is you can definitely still satisfy the food cravings you have by choosing better options that are simple to implement and easy to live with long term, and that's what makes it so effective in replacing your old diet with new healthier habits.

Time magazine had a really interesting issue titled "The Weight Loss Trap: Why your diet isn't working," and one of the articles in it that jumped out at me was about the show *The Biggest Loser*. I'll summarize here: Kevin Hall, a scientist with the National Institute of Health, started watching the show after a friend suggested he check it out. Kevin tuned in and saw that these contestants were, in fact, showing some big drops when they stepped on the scale for the weekly weigh-in . . . 20 lbs. a week was not uncommon. In fact, the average contestant lost 127 lbs. during the entire season and about 64% of their body fat. Kevin was interested enough in what was going on there to research and write a paper on it featuring 14 of the contestants. During the research, Kevin found that 13 of the 14 contestants gained an average of 66% of their weight back and four gained weight that made them heavier than before they went on the show. While the show created an ideal environment built for weight loss—tailor-made meal plans, motivating trainers, prizes, a staff of doctors—without that structure in place at home, the weight came back. The plan they were following, which was created for the length of the show taping, simply wasn't sustainable. What it came down to was that once the external support resources were removed, the contestants did not have their own process in place to rely on every day. So why does this always seem to happen with diets . . . why is it so hard to keep weight off (assuming it was lost to begin with)? This question has no simple answer, which is why people have been searching for and selling ideas about it for a very long time. With the majority of Americans falling into the category of overweight or obese and the corresponding health (and healthcare cost) implications being so dire, there is a continuous quest to address and help slow this epidemic.

One of these measures came in the form of a $930 million study funded by the NIH (which is part of what Kevin was writing his paper for), and one of its main objectives was to see what was working and what wasn't. When you get down to the bottom line, that's the holy grail of any study into weight loss . . . what works and stays working. Any study that costs $930 million is going to result in mountains of data which will not be covered here, but one of the key takeaway points is that in various groups there was a percentage of people that had consistent success with diet plans and the universal theme involved changing lifestyle habits, not simply what they ate or didn't eat.

In the same spirit of trying to determine what works long term, the National Weight Control Registry (NWCR) invited people to participate in their study if you met certain criteria; specifically, having lost 30 lbs. and keeping it off for at least a year. Over the past 25 years that it has been going on, the list has grown to over 10,000 people from all 50 states who have lost an average of 66 lbs. for over five years. Of that group some of the most common traits attributed to success are: adding some form of exercise into their weekly routine (daily walking ranked highest), weighing themselves weekly, limiting daily television hours, removing junk food from their house, keeping a food journal, and limiting portion size. These behavioral changes were all shared, regardless of the actual food being eaten. This shows the significant and time-tested effectiveness of finding changes that are manageable and very meaningful in bringing permanent changes that result in new habits.

Each of us has different priorities and objectives when it comes to our diet during BAR40, but in general there are two areas that tend to be of highest interest. One would be improving the quality of what you eat with the goal of enjoying the longest life possible and at peak fitness levels. The other goal tends to be achieving your optimal weight, which will help you look and feel your best, and of course, has the added bonus of improving your overall health in all of the areas you're likely already familiar with. A third category would be that you already live by a diet that you consider perfect for you and you are completely happy to maintain your current weight without adding or losing a pound. If that's you, then well done and keep up the awesome work! For the majority of us, though, determining the best food choices takes some work and periodic adjustments. Not surprisingly, like almost every other imaginable topic, the internet brings an endless supply of information, much of it conflicting. To save you time in hunting through a lot of online nonsense, I'll pass along two suggestions you may want to take a look at.

One is the USDA site and in particular, the current edition of the Dietary Guidelines for Americans (DGA). Starting in 1990, this is something that the government requires to be published every five years, and the current one is the 2015-2020 edition. I know the idea of government food guidelines may bring back memories from the 5th grade and posters in the cafeteria of a glass of milk with an apple but keep an open mind until you check it out. Unlike some areas of the government that seem to be frozen in time, destined to bureaucratic groundhog days . . . the USDA has done an impressive job tackling a tough topic with a ton of moving parts.

For example, the current guidelines booklet (144-page PDF ready for download or print at dietaryguidelines.gov) had an overhaul since the previous edition. Basically, as you can read in the Executive Summary, there was a realization that the guidelines were (I'm paraphrasing here) out of touch based on feedback from the advisory committee and public comments. Factoring in those reviews, the focus of the current edition has been revamped to reflect how people actually eat in America. Instead of separate data analytics of the major food groups, the current resource looks at what is referred to as "food patterns," or simply put . . . how we combine different foods when we make meals and ways to do it better.

Another aspect that I like about the current DGA is that it has an emphasis on food "shifts," which is their way of talking about improvements through substitution. Last but not least on why I think the USDA site is worth a visit . . . check out the MyPlate feature (you can also go directly there at choosemyplate.gov). It's a quick and easy tool that creates a (somewhat) customized food plan based on your age, sex, weight, height, and activity level. It breaks your daily requirements down by group and meal (fruit, veggie, protein, etc.) and converts it to a PDF for printing, which puts it into a food journal format where you can check boxes, add comments, or make notes. It's a pretty slick resource that you may find useful . . . I'd say it's free, but technically, we already paid for it in some small way through federal taxes if you're reading this in the US!

The other recommendation I have for you as an awesome nutrition and healthy eating book is *On Target Living* by Chris Johnson. I first got this book in 2011 (it was actually an assigned text in a class I was taking on mindfulness), and I've referred to it often in the years since then. This book is all about how we maximize our performance potential in life through optimal nutrition. It not only talks about how important the quality of fuel in our engine is, but it's packed with tips, tools, shopping lists, meal plans and resources that cover any possible question that you will have when it comes to building your best personalized diet. I can say without any doubt that this book is what got me started on the substitution approach of looking at what you're eating and just making it a little better.

Another part of the book I found to be an enormous help

is the Food Target tool, which is available for free download on the *On Target Living* site. I included a photo of it on the next page, so you get an idea of what I'm describing but do yourself a favor and print out the actual PDF or order the larger laminated version from the site. I have had that Food Target on our refrigerator door for years (literally), and I see it every day. It does a great job of providing "good, better, best" options for a ton of different foods, but it also serves as a frequent daily reminder to try and incrementally improve what you're eating. Remember . . . the best diet is the one that works for you. Words of wisdom from the $930 million dollar study.

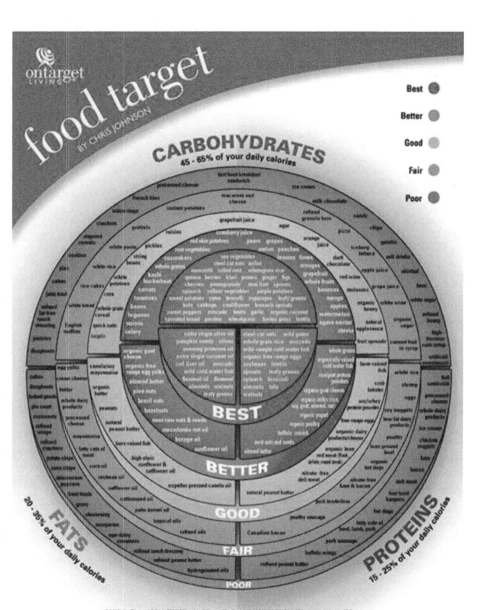

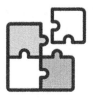

Mindset

S teve Jobs had a great quote, "If you really look closely, most overnight successes took a long time." One of the most important and valuable parts of BAR40, and one that will stay with you long after the 52 weeks is done is the achievement mindset. While exercise and diet improvements are major components of this program, the mental training aspect is the real engine that's driving the train and is by far the most powerful aspect that will have the most significant impacts in every area of your life. Why I like that Steve Jobs quote is that I think it hits the nail on the head with regard to the pursuit of personal excellence and self-mastery. When it comes to becoming the best, most successful version of yourself, it is a lifetime pursuit, there are no two ways about it. Simply put, there is no finish line. Time is constantly moving us forward through life, and each day, we have an abundance of small choices to make, like small forks in the road. One way will slightly elevate or improve us, and the other is bringing us slightly down. In its individual form the decision, either way, is probably inconsequential. "I'm supposed to exercise today, but I don't feel like it" is a perfect example as it's something that anyone fitness-oriented has experienced. If you skip working out nothing terrible happens, and if you do work out nothing amazing or awesome instantly happens . . . either decision brings no noticeable outcome in the immediate sense. The choice to procrastinate brings us slightly down as we take the easy way out and ever so slightly add a little fuel to the subconscious habit equation formula of, skipping a workout is fine when _____ (fill in the blank with the excuse of choice). On the other hand, the harder decision to do the workout and tough it out is one more opportunity to subconsciously reinforce the notion that self-commitments are going to be upheld and procrastination is not an option. It gives us one more small chance to get more comfortable being uncomfortable and build that muscle of mental toughness and resilience. Although this is one mundane "typical Tuesday" example, there are these types of small crossroads continuously presenting themselves not only with regard to diet and exercise but relationships with our family and friends, career choices, and financial decisions.

Almost every aspect of our life comes with sets of small choices and creating the habit of continuously taking the slightly higher road is constantly pointing the trajectory of your life at an upward angle. Conversely, the habit of taking the easy road is setting your course at a downward angle and subconsciously creating the habit that the default choice is the slightly easier "maybe tomorrow" option.

As Dale Carnegie puts it, "Today is the tomorrow you worried about yesterday."

The more we can get into the habit of living each day to the best of our abilities, making the slightly better, tougher choice in those small instances that pop up throughout the day you will find that you are in fact living the "best day ever" approach which is going to bring you to your best year ever. Once again we can look at the principle of compounding, but instead of your interest earning interest and accelerating financial wealth, it's your daily habit of making the tougher, better choices which are building upon the foundation of all of your yesterdays that have been continuously angling your life's trajectory upwards.

Without question, there is an enormous number of self-help and personal improvement books that have been written over the years, and a lot of them make promises geared toward overnight success, quick fixes, and overly simple solutions to life's complex problems. Common sense tells us any promise of results with no effort is nonsense, but more importantly, it brings to light the underlying and fundamental challenge that we all face every day. We tend to live in societies that are accustomed to instant gratification. Our 2020 world is geared toward "on demand" fulfillment: we get what we want, when we want it. While that brings all sorts of convenience with regard to shopping, watching TV, and food delivery, it's counter to the daily practice of delayed gratification. Essentially, working harder today to make our tomorrow better.

While BAR40 is not a magic wand approach that will suddenly and miraculously make you the best version of yourself overnight, the daily practices will create the mindset that will help reach your full potential. I've included some key components that I practice in my daily life that I have found to be highly beneficial over the years in helping provide the framework and structure for continuous progress.

Get Acquainted with your Future Self

How often do you hear someone say (perhaps you) that they wish they could tell their younger self to do or not do something? It's human nature; we tend to Monday morning quarterback things with the wisdom of hindsight and think of what we could have done differently. This, as we know but often overlook, is a pointless exercise that does absolutely no good. At best, that tendency to dwell in the past with the would have/ could have/should have/ self-talk regret is a waste of time, but worse, it distracts you from the current situation and clouds your thought process. In recognizing the fact that we all have the tendency to want to offer words of wisdom via time travel, we can still satisfy that impulse, but we just need to adjust the timeline. Think of it this way: we can still offer advice to our younger self; all we have to do is start thinking in terms of the future you. For example, If you're 50 years old now, instead of thinking about what you would do if you had the chance to go back 15 years and re-do life choices you made at 35 years old, adjust the timeline. Visualize yourself at 65 years old and think about what you would say to yourself at 50. Really make the effort to imagine yourself 15 years from now and think about what you wish you could have done differently, what passions you would have pursued, what decisions you would have made differently, what health and fitness choices you wish you would have put into place and stuck with.

This approach may sound a little out there in concept, but I can't encourage you strongly enough to try and incorporate it into your daily outlook. This form of mental time travel is already wired into our thought process in the sense that we tend to think in terms of what could have been done differently, except by shifting the time frame forward we are harnessing this way of thinking into a very productive tool. It's easy to use the example of the old and infirm CEO on his deathbed, more money than he could ever spend sitting in his various accounts, pledging he would give it all up just to have one month with his kids again when they were young. While that one may be a common cliché, it does speak to the fact that if we are able to recognize in real-time what's most important without needing the lens of retrospect, we are able to make decisions that better serve our real priorities. It's like in *A Christmas Carol* when Ebenezer Scrooge has the visit from the ghost of Christmas future and has a vision of how his life turns out (spoiler if you haven't seen it . . . it's not a great outcome for Scrooge). Scrooge wakes up to find himself back in the present day with a chance to change his ways, alter the course he was on, and avoid the future that awaited him in the vision. The idea is to appreciate the good old days while they are occurring in real-time instead of when they're long gone.

So strike up a friendship with your future self, open up the lines of communication and instead of thinking about what you would do differently then . . . think about what you should do differently now. Being in the habit of letting your future self provide guidance on your current decisions will have a profound impact on avoiding all the easy short-term choices that are at odds with your long-term goals.

The notion of the two selves (present and future) is an area that has drawn plenty of attention and research over the years, in particular as it relates to retirement planning. This is a perfect example of the two selves at odds with each other. Our present self thinks buying a new Corvette is a great idea; the future self strongly disagrees and votes for putting that money into retirement savings. Our future self is shouting from a distance, so the voice is easily drowned out by the loud and close enthusiasm of our present self, which may be why the present self wins the coin toss so frequently. An interesting TED Talk you can check out on the topic is by Daniel Goldstein back in 2011, and in it he talks about a study using a "Behavioral Time Machine." To sum it up, the main challenge for a lot of people in creating a dialogue with their future self is that they consider that person a stranger, and in having that disconnected feeling toward them, their needs warrant a lesser priority than their present self. Because of this mental blind spot our future self tends to constantly live in a disadvantaged position unless we actively change that behavior. This Time Machine experiment is based on the research that our neural patterns are much different when there are visual cues versus just imagining our future self. Based on that, it showed participants digitally aged avatars of themselves complete with various emotional responses based on their financial position in relation to current savings rates. For example: saving now shows the future monthly retirement fund growing and your older self beginning to look happier. Less money later, and future you starts looking downright angry! The big deal about the test is that it showed conclusive results that a "future self" image could visually knock some sense into our present self brain and change our decision making to deliver better long-term outcomes. Beyond financial planning, they have experimented with ethical decisions, academic performance, and weight loss. I bring this experiment up as an additional tool to think about if you are having difficulty in getting the mindset of fast-forwarding through time. There are free apps and websites available that will age your uploaded selfie and even show different versions of it based on choices and changes you can make (smoking and sun exposure, for example).

With or without the visual tools to help . . . develop the habit of making your future self proud!

As I write this, I think about an example this week where I was about to go out for a run, and my 10-year-old daughter, Riley, wanted me to go for a bike ride with her. My first impulse was to say that I couldn't go because I was about to go running. But after years of practicing what I preach with regard to the future self, my thoughts recalibrated to the fact that the opportunity to go for a bike ride with my 10-year-old daughter was a finite moment in time I should not miss, versus my run, which would be pretty much the same as yesterday's and tomorrow's.

Would life be much different either way, whether I went on the bike ride or didn't go? Of course not, life would have pretty much gone on as normal either way, but I know that I never want to look back with regret and the thought that if I could just go back to age 44 and say to myself, Hey dummy, take the bike ride with Riley . . . she may not be asking you to do that when she's a teenager.

EQ

Being in continuous communication with your future self, as useful as the practice is, in no way lessens the importance of optimizing your day-to-day to performance. Further developing the emotional skill sets that allow you to best deal with any situation that comes up is a pursuit that pays enormous dividends and one that we, at least here in the US, do not always give a lot of thought to (nor do we typically see it on our kids' curriculum at school, unfortunately).

We all come equipped with this amazing human technology component, our brain, that has enormous power and potential but no instruction manual on how to use it. As an example of how much firepower we're carrying around with us, the University of California-Berkeley devised a computation program to measure the speed and calculating capability of a normal functioning brain and compared it to the IBM Sequoia, the world's most advanced artificial intelligence supercomputer at the time of the 2015 study. IBM developed the Sequoia for the National Nuclear Security Administration in 2011, at a cost of about $250 million, and while it was still the most advanced computer in the world, the study results showed that the human brain was approximately 30 times faster at shifting data around. They also went on to point out that if we were able to rent out brain's computing power and charge the same thousands of dollars per hour that the Sequoia billed, brain renting would be the universally preferred side hustle.

So we're born with this incredible tool but mainly are left to our own devices to figure out how it works when it comes to all of the emotions and feelings that are constantly being generated. There has been a growing trend in the past few years toward living more mindfully, but what does that mean exactly? Similar to diets, this is a topic that plenty of books have been written about and cutting through the mountains of research posted online to determine the best approach with maximum benefit is where my objective is.

One of the areas that I found to be most useful in learning more about over the years is emotional intelligence, or EQ as it's become more commonly known. As a one-sentence summary, EQ is the ability to rapidly recognize emotions in yourself and others and deal with them most appropriately. There is perhaps no better example of a "simple but not easy" concept than that one but developing these skills around self-management deliver far-reaching results not only in your life but also those around you. If there is any type of "owner's manual" for the mind, I would suspect it would be based around the four concepts of emotional intelligence: self-awareness, self-management, social awareness, and relationship management.

First, let's consider how the brain is hardwired so we can better understand the default setting on that supercomputer of ours. All of our senses, everything we touch, taste, see, smell, and hear, move through our body in the form of electric signals which enter our brain through the spinal cord. The final destination of all of these electric signals is the frontal lobe, where they are converted into rational thoughts. Prior to reaching the frontal lobe, though, all of those signals pass through the limbic system, which is the place where emotional responses are created/felt. So think about that for a second: before our brain has a chance to rationally process the information coming in, there has already been an emo- tional reaction to it. Emotional intelligence in its physical form is basically the communication between the two very important processing centers: the emotions (limbic system) and rational thoughts (frontal lobe). The more effective the communication process is, the better we are able to manage our emotions. The implications for this are far-reaching as it relates to the spectrum of life successes, including every-thing from how we interact in personal and professional relationships to career and financial gain. In general terms, EQ significantly shapes how we are perceived by others every day, which is a big reason why it continues to gain momentum and attention as a field of study.

Ever since *Time* magazine featured emotional intelligence as a cover story and debated whether it was more important than IQ as a predictor of future success, it has been an area of intense focus.

Another big reason for the high level of interest in EQ is the comparison to IQ and what the differences can mean. IQ is understood to be a set point . . . we get what we get in life and play the hand we're dealt. The accepted theory is that our IQ at age 16 is the same at 66. EQ, on the other hand, is not set at a fixed point and is something we can actively work at developing and improving. It's not surprising that there is a lot of controversy and debate on the topic.

To oversimplify the whole thing, we can take two people and try to guess who will find more success using established criteria for their field in the same given job. One scores "high IQ/average EQ" and the other "high EQ/average IQ." Let's say that IQ relates to "hard skills" like becoming a brain surgeon, and EQ relates to "soft skills" like being able to use intuition to read a situation and respond accordingly. Conventional wisdom would say that the smart money is on the person with high IQ reaching higher levels of success than Person 2 with the higher EQ, but it's not that simple. Data shows that there are plenty of people with a high IQ that are surpassed by colleagues in the same field with a lower IQ but higher EQ. While there are thousands of pages of research, reports, and findings, we don't have to look any further than the people we know in our own lives to have a clear understanding of how that happens. You may work with someone who is generally considered a super genius rocket scientist type with more technical knowledge than anybody (just ask him and he'll tell you), but the problem is that he is a complete nightmare to be around. He's just one of those toxic people that never misses a chance to say something condescending or belittles your contribution to a project you're both working on or is just a generally abrasive personality type to be around. In some way or another, he (we'll make this villain male) has managed to insult everyone in the office at some point, and he makes no secret about the fact that he does not care; he's there to do his job, not make friends. On the other side of the office is another person on the same team that's competent in technical knowledge and does her job as expected. In addition, though, her upbeat attitude, quick wit, genuine interest, and affection toward her coworkers and all-around positive energy make her arrival into any room a reason to become a little happier and ultimately leaves people in a better mood after spending any time around her.

This example shows opposite ends of the spectrum, but I'm guessing you can relate to these types of people based on your own work experience, and I would bet that in most cases that Person 2 is going to go further, faster than Person 1. Person 2, in all likelihood, has a high level of self-awareness that translates into all-around likability. These traits generally include being optimistic, authentic, using other people's names, positive body language, generally easy to be around, and have the sort of magnetic personality that draws people into wanting to be in their orbit.

Why I consider EQ to be such an important area for us to be mindful of developing every day is that in some way or another it impacts all areas in our life, starting with our own thoughts and emotions. To get back to the earlier point on the input from our senses becoming converted into feelings before they have a chance to have rational thought applied . . . that's a major area for potential improvement that we can work on every day.

Here are some ideas and areas that I think will be of use to you:

Emotional observation — The problem with feelings becoming emotions before rational thought is applied is that we automatically react to something before we have a chance to think about it. Unless it's one of the very rare true fight or flight moments in your life, then thinking before acting and reacting is the better choice. The act of making a conscious effort to notice emotions as they are bubbling up, being witness to them instead of being a passenger as they take control of the wheel. Taking that moment of pause and recognizing the feeling allows the rational thought to be applied to the emotion and prevents you from simply reacting.

For example, you're at a red light driving to work, distracted by an urgent email that you saw pop up on your phone. While you're looking down at it, the light turns green, and the guy behind you hits the horn for a little longer than necessary to get your attention. We've all been there, whether the honker or honked at. Our immediate natural response is probably some sort of anger . . . Hey, calm down _____ (pick your name)! which is our fight response being activated. We drive away, muttering under our breath and thinking dark thoughts about that other driver and his hopefully imminent death, maybe respond with a finger, and then we think about it for a while afterward and take the distraction into work with us.

That single brief moment could have a ripple effect that not only puts you in a bad mood for the morning but in some slight way influences how you treat your coworkers and in turn impacts their mood . . . right down the line it goes. This is the type of emotional hijacking that you can train yourself to avoid and stop all that negativity in its tracks, by taking that moment of pause, identifying that the feeling of anger is there, and making the choice not to react to it. You can't help what feelings come up; you can only help how you react to them. Put another way, you can be a witness to your emotions without allowing them to dictate your actions. This deals with the self-awareness component of EQ, developing the habit to observe yourself in real-time, objectively, with the intention of identifying areas you want to change.

That said, sometimes our efforts at self-awareness can only take us so far as they have limitations based on our own baked-in perspectives, biases, and in general, the lens we see everything through. Getting candid feedback from the people we trust in our life on how we are perceived is always useful, assuming you're able to get past the fact that there will be some discomfort in hearing things that are contrary to how we see ourselves. Think of when we hear our own voice in a video or on a voicemail. There tends to be that thought of, I don't really sound like that! The same thing is going on all the time with how we come across to others. We simply do not always know how we are perceived by other people. A couple of years back, my company did an anonymous 360-assessment in the form of start/stop/continue feedback. At the end of it, everyone got a brief summary of constructive feedback. One thing that jumped out at me was the fact that most people thought I talked way too fast and that I should slow it down to more effectively communicate information when I was doing presentations. While it's a fairly minor critique, it was something I never considered, yet it was something that just about everyone else I worked with pointed out as an area for improvement. Based on that feedback I became more mindful of how fast I was speaking, and in turn, I began to notice a higher level of feedback and questions at the end of presentations which suggests that prior to slowing things down, not all of the material I was presenting was delivered in a way that was being absorbed.

Self-management is the aspect of EQ that deals with your awareness and puts the rubber to the road with tools and actions. It's more than simply recognizing you're becoming extremely frustrated at your spouse and stifling the impulse to shout about it. (Although the self-stifling tends to be a good plan too!) These practices and habits incorporated into your daily life will go a long way toward bringing significant benefits not only to you but those around you.

Breathing techniques—Think of all the movies when someone is overly excited, panicked, or frazzled and the response they get is "calm down, take a breath!" While that may not be something you put into practice in your own life, it's definitely worth doing. Using breathing techniques is the ultimate secret weapon in regulating your own emotions during feelings of stress or in any situation without anyone even knowing you're doing it. It really is like the reset button for your brain. Give it a try right now. Inhale four seconds through your nose, hold it for a second, four second exhalation through your mouth and repeat a few times. Automatically you feel a little calmer; it slows time down and gives a quick boost of clarity. This can be done anytime and never seems to lose its effectiveness. It's also helpful for staying focused in conversations with other people and helps you concentrate on what the other person is saying and overrides our natural tendency to be thinking about what we are going to say next as opposed to what is being said. Being a better active listener instead of "reloading" while we wait to talk again is a highly worthwhile pursuit.

Another technique and one actively used by military Special Ops teams is "box breathing." This is a remarkable stress management approach that once again, you can put to use any time you feel pressure rising and want to put the brakes on your emotions. In this exercise, you visualize a square and start at the lower-left corner. Inhale for four seconds while going up the left side of the box. Hold your breath for four seconds while you visualize going across the top. Next, exhale for four seconds as you go down the right side. Lastly, hold your breath for four seconds as you cross the bottom back to where you started. The whole trip around takes 16 seconds, so in roughly a minute, you will have gone around the box four times, and the calming effects are well worth the time. Again, give it a try and see for yourself. Doing it with your eyes closed helps with the box visualization and tends to have more of a relaxing effect, but you can certainly do it with your eyes open. I can't imagine Navy SEALS that are doing this in combat situations always have the option of closing their eyes, so we know it works either way!

Set aside time for a daily review — You'll find that in the daily training journal pages, there's a place to make note of each day's highlights. Spending a few minutes every day to reflect on what went right and what could have gone better is a habit that helps distill the 24 hours down into the major headlines. Something that you make note of wishing you had done differently today becomes a tangible goal to implement tomorrow. It also is a place to record successes and milestones . . . "catch yourself doing something right" as the saying goes. Having a routine of recording three or four daily successes will also make you more mindful throughout the day of doing things that you'll be putting on that list later on. If you're the type of person who sets personal goals and holds yourself accountable to them, then this is a great additional way to get you thinking throughout the day . . . where am I on my list today? I don't have any doubt you will easily reach the daily three noteworthy successes, but the fact that you are taking the step to record them every day will automatically bump them up in your daily prioritization and help ensure you are always looking through the lens of what can be done above and beyond how you may normally do something. Again, the best year ever is made up of 365 best days and this helps serve that purpose.

This daily journal and review are something only you will

see, so take the opportunity to review openly and honestly what's working and what needs improvement.

Get better at being present in the present — This is a tough area for all of us above the age of 10 years old it seems, and with more kids having phones now that age is probably getting younger! The concept is simple enough: when we're thinking about what went on yesterday or last week or planning the thousand things that need to be done for work and on the home to-do list, our mental focus is dragged back or pulled forward. No matter how good we think we are at mental multitasking, it's almost as tough to be in two places at once mentally as it is to be physically. The main reason I have for encouraging you to add this as a priority to your daily mental training is that by shifting your focus to the here and now, you are able to get in the habit of really experiencing all of the great things that are going on each day. Once again, the concept here is to appreciate the "good old days" while they're happening instead of the common alternative of looking back on memories and appreciating them after they have passed us by. If you're able to get into the mindset of experiencing events fully while they're going on, you're going to have a much different level of appreciation for the good stuff and also be better equipped to manage and deal with any of the negative aspects that pop up. While I don't see how "live every day like it's your last" can realistically be put to use in the literal sense, I definitely think a modified version of "live your days like they are few but live life like it's endless" is an approach that can definitely work for you. While we all need to plan for the future, that doesn't mean we shouldn't be making every day matter. It's not a one or the other option; both trains can run simultaneously on parallel tracks. The optimal middle ground includes having a clear vision on where you want to see your life go and how to best direct it toward the desired outcomes, but it also allows for making the most of every single day with the realization that there is never a guaranteed tomorrow. I realize this sort of idea can come across as cliché, but if you actively start making it a practice to corral your thoughts and isolate them to the present, you will without question see how easy and effective it can be toward improving your effectiveness at whatever you're doing as well as the actual enjoyment and appreciation of it.

This week try this visualization approach and see if it works for you. Imagine you're writing your life's story and every day is a brand-new blank page in the book waiting to be filled up. (Go all in, imagine the actual book . . . leather-bound, gold leaf pages, a red bookmark . . . whatever you want your book to look like!) The future is entirely unwritten, just open pages. The previous chapters are written, of course, but history is not destiny, and what happens in the rest of the book is still up to you. If you give thought to what events you want to include in the story, you can structure the plot to start heading in that direction. Knowing the end of the story isn't the goal; unexpected plot twists will bring plenty of future zigging and zagging from your original plan but having some main story points to aim for will at least let you navigate in that direction. Another way to look at it: think of it as if you were the subject of a movie. There is no rehearsal in this life of ours; it's a live production, and the cameras are rolling! Think about your future self again with the question being: what can I be doing to avoid any regrets down the road on what I wished I did more of and what I should have prioritized? There's a lot of truth to the expression that "life is what happens when you're busy making other plans." Just think about how easy it is to plan for a summer vacation, look forward to the trip for months and when we finally find ourselves on that vacation we're checking our phone and thinking about what needs to be done when we get back. I get it, that dedication and task-oriented mindset is a big part of your success and is not something that can be turned off. That said, if you are able to build the skills that allow you to refine your focus and compartmentalize the distractions from taking away from your being fully present in the given moment, then you develop the skill set to make the most of it. As Mark Twain wrote, "Worrying about the future is like paying a debt we don't owe."

Become the CEO of your life — Years ago, I read an article about an approach to managing your life like it was a company, and the idea has stayed with me and proved to be very useful in becoming more objective about decision making. Try this experiment, and I think you'll find it's not difficult to see the similarities between our lives and any Fortune 100 company. Imagine you are the CEO of a large and profitable organization . . . "You, Inc." There are many people involved both as employees and shareholders, competing goals, multiple departments and business units, daily challenges and uncertainties, and a never-ending to-do list competing for your attention that needs prioritization. As CEO, sitting back and letting whatever is going to happen just go ahead and happen is simply not an option that will lead to success. Strategic thinking and practices need to become a foundation of how your company operates across all the departments. As the Chief Executive, you have the final responsibility to make sure things are happening in ways that are in concert with your ultimate vision. As the saying goes, "heavy is the head that wears the crown," and when you're in that top seat the buck stops with you.

While we have talented and trusted people around us that we rely on to help ensure objectives are accomplished, we, as CEOs, are the ones that have to set the overall course and constantly lead the company toward success.

While all of those things are true for a CEO, they are also true for your own life. For example, instead of different "departments" we have habits that we need to keep an eye on to make sure they are performing in ways that support the big picture. While there may not be "company policies" in our life, the various habits we have, both good and bad, end up being the default way we run our company every day. I find this to be the main benefit of envisioning yourself as the CEO. It allows you to objectively look at things through the lens of what you would do in the context of your business. Here are some areas and outlooks I have put into place over the years that I find to be most beneficial:

Who are the people in your company? This works whether you have your CEO hat on or in the context of the company you keep. There is no getting around the fact that the people we spend the most time with us have a significant impact and influence on us whether we realize it or not. This can be a huge benefit to us or a force that works against us, acting as a headwind that slows us down or, worse, points us in the wrong direction. No doubt you have heard some version of the expression "birds of a feather flock together" or "show me your friends and I'll tell you who you are" but there is plenty of research on the subject that shows conclusive evidence of the long term impacts in either direction that the people we spend the most time with have on our lives. For me, this means that I limit my time around what I consider "toxic personality types" to as little as possible. I'm not a smoker, so I would no more sit in a closed room with a chain-smoker breathing in their second-hand smoke than I would spend time with people that have an emotional outlook that is permanently set in the negative spectrum. Everyone has bad days, of course; I'm not talking about that. What I'm referring to are the people who are always the victim ("bad things always happen to me"), overly judgmental (always quick to tell you what's right or wrong), the pessimist (on a sunny day they'll tell you it's supposed to rain tomorrow), gossip obsessed (they quickly steer every conversation to something starting with, did you hear . . .), the self-absorbed (if the conversation isn't about them then they're mentally checked out or finding a way to bring it back to them), and the constantly jealous. Having frequent and prolonged time spent around these sorts of conversations and personality types is doing you absolutely no favors in becoming the best version of yourself, and my suggestion would be finding ways to limit that exposure to as little as possible. We will always have coworkers and even family members who fall into these categories, and while we aren't going to write them off in life, we can definitely be mindful of those traits and not get sucked into the vortex of being drawn into that negative energy field more often than necessary.

Thinking of it from the CEO perspective, would you want employees in your company that were constantly complaining and generally negative people bringing that negativity around other employees every day and dragging morale down? Alternatively, building teams that are made up of people focused on ideas and innovation help create a culture of positivity and achievement that is contagious throughout the organization. Whether it's your circle of influence in your personal life or using the example of your company, it's an easy choice on what sort of group is going to deliver the biggest positive impact.

Growth versus fixed mindset is an interesting area that has received a lot of attention in academic settings on how we teach kids, but this is something we can definitely apply in our adult lives every day. To simplify the concept, we are all born with a disposition that leans one way or the other. We can look at any circumstance and say this is the way it is (fixed), or we can see it as something we have the power to change (growth). Dr. Carol Dweck is credited with being one of the leading pioneers in this field and cast a lot of light on an area that was not previously explored to great lengths, although it is now thought to be a fundamental factor in how we deal with challenges and failure and how we pursue our goals. There is an abundance of research information available based on the neuroscience discoveries around brain plasticity and neural networks being more malleable than previously known (and it's worth a Google look), but I find the most important point to be that the research is conclusive in that a growth mindset leads to increased success and achievements and, even better, it's an area we can improve. Throughout the studies that Dweck and her teams did, the evidence clearly showed that for the students classified as "fixed mindset" it was entirely possible to change and retrain the brain, which showed new brain growth and increased speed in neural transmission previously thought to be impossible.

For me, this comes back to the idea of looking at things we do throughout each day through the lens of "is this the best I can do?" Getting into this habit, which is basically the constant pursuit of personal excellence, is a major factor in creating the habit of constant improvement. This is not to say that all things you do every waking minute are going to be at 110%; that's not realistic or sustainable. More to the point is that you are creating a thought pattern in yourself that you are automatically looking at a small way to do whatever it is you're doing just a little bit better.

When you look at the fixed versus growth mindset in the context as CEO of your company, it's easy to see pick out the businesses that operate with the philosophy "we do it this way because this is the way we have always done it." Those companies are easy to spot because they don't often survive!

Let's go back to the Food Target I mentioned earlier in talking about diet. If you like eating ice cream but don't like the calories, sugar, and fat that go along with it, then do it better. Have low-fat frozen yogurt and still satisfy the craving but in an improved way that works long term. This same concept can be applied to everything you're doing. In a conversation with a coworker, could you be listening more instead of letting your mind wander? Are you going to let yourself skip a workout because it may rain, or are you going to stick to the plan and do it? Are you practicing awareness of what your emotional state is and recognizing feelings without being hijacked by them? When you're having a conversation with your young son or daughter are you recognizing the opportunity to develop your patience and self-management by letting them tell some meandering, never-ending story about a dream they had about a purple bird instead of cutting it short because it's a ridiculous story with no point and you have more important things to do?

Get gritty — Grit is often described as perseverance plus passion and, to me, is one of the most underrated secret weapons out there that will help make you unstoppable in your efforts. Developing or strengthening this mental toughness and creating the deep belief in yourself that failure is not an option is going to automatically remove the escape hatches that prevent you from doing what you know is the best, but often the hardest thing to do. Maybe one of the best expressions that captures the essence of this daily outlook is "burn the boats." While the origin may be with commanders in battle issuing orders to destroy the ships, leaving only victory or death as the possible outcomes, we can put this to use in life every day by focusing only on what needs to be done and how we are going to do it in order to succeed. Putting an end to thought patterns about reasons why something won't work and getting rid of the unfounded self-doubts that take away from your potential is a huge step toward building an ironclad mental resilience.

This will not only allow you to achieve what you are setting out to do, it will create the competitive drive in you that has you looking for extra challenges around every corner just for the chance at one more opportunity for another victory of some sort!

Problems and challenges are always going to come up; we all know there is no getting around that fact. While there is no point in trying to avoid all of the unexpected events that are often out of our control in life, the one thing we can definitely control is our skill sets in dealing with the challenges. In building our mental toughness to hit the challenges head-on, we become much better at handling them with the approach of "identify, adapt and evolve." Having this daily mindset of self-confidence means that whatever comes your way is something that you can break down into parts and manage without being overwhelmed.

Think about people in your life that no matter what the crisis, they are the people you know would have a solution and would be able to deal with it. Maybe it's a friend, family member, neighbor, or coworker, but no matter who, if World War III broke out, they are someone you would want by your side in the foxhole. This person does not have any superpower, obviously, but it's very likely that they have built up the skills and mentality over time that they can handle anything that life throws at them and come out of it tougher, stronger, and learn something new in the process.

While this is not an overnight transformation, the daily discipline and attitude will be bringing incremental changes every day. Even if you don't notice an immediate change, when you stick with it for the duration of BAR40 I have no doubt whatsoever that your resilience, drive, determination, and willingness to accept defeat will have undergone a massive transformation.

Another major factor in this increasing self-assuredness is that outside negativity from the people we can't avoid will cease to have any impact on your momentum. Ultimately it comes down to the perspective that I don't have any problem with someone telling me why some challenge can't be done as long as they don't get in my way while I'm doing it.

Having the drive to identify what you want to do and the determination to do it is something many others around you will not have. Simply put, getting comfortable being uncomfortable and doing what others can't or won't do will make you an outlier in the sense that you are building a framework for life that always involves going that one extra step and being in the habit of putting in that small extra effort.

In my experience, it's often as basic as the fact that successful people are willing to do what unsuccessful people are not willing to do . . . every day and in almost every way.

As the CEO of your company, when you think about what it's going to take to continuously succeed and be an industry leader, consider those traits of perseverance, a focus on best-practices, determination, and a company philosophy of constant improvement. It's a simple, but not easy, recipe for success.

A lot of this can once again be put in the context of making your future self proud and the idea of delayed gratification. Every one of us gets the same 168 hours each week to put to use, and how we allocate those hours is where paths diverge in very different directions. I think of time in two different ways.

There's time . . . and there is our Time. The first time is how we spend our days, those are the hours we get every day. The second one is our Time, meaning what we did with our life on this planet. How we choose to spend our time is ultimately how we spent our Time in that our "today" is built on all of those accumulated yesterdays. This is directly tied into the idea of BAR40 being the best year ever by way of 365 chances of living your best day, getting rid of procrastination, and creating daily habits to take the extra steps to improve and elevate yourself. Think about all the small things that you do each day and if/how they can be done better.

Drinking

Last but not least . . . let's talk about (not) drinking! As I alluded to back in the Introduction, this aspect of BAR40 can evoke an immediate and dug in, arms crossed, head shaking, flat out refusal by plenty of people who are simply not interested in parting ways with alcohol for a year. If you're in that category, then by all means, feel free to skip this section. I have no axe to grind against alcohol and am not on any crusade to rid the world of the "the devil's drink" once and for all! Trying to convince someone to stop drinking who truly does not want to stop is a fool's errand that I have no desire to spend time attempting. My only intent is to provide some background and information on why I consider removing alcohol to be a major advantage in realizing the full potential of your best year ever.

Also, while I know there are a certain percentage of people that are dead set against giving up drinking, I also realize there's an equally significant percentage of you that are sober-curious (to use the increasingly popular 2021 term) or want to quit drinking altogether and have not found the right time or way to do that yet. If you are in this second category, then I think you will find that BAR40 is the perfect time and place to give the non-drinking life a test drive.

As for a little background on the "dry" aspect of BAR40, it goes back to when I was 39 and thinking about what my 40th "best year ever" would entail and specifically, what the main differences from my normal routine would be. I was putting together the ideas of what would eventually become BAR40, and in looking at the main areas of improvement, I could see pretty quickly that my fondness for drinking beer was in direct conflict with virtually every goal I had. First off, I knew I wanted to lose weight and realized that a lot of my daily calories were coming from beer. Not to mention that pub food and late-night eating were also part of the problem. I was also thinking about how I wanted to maximize my productivity every day and thought about how often I felt tired on the weekends after a bunch of beers and the resulting poor sleep.

When it came to exercise, when I looked at my running journal and isolated the days that I skipped running, cut it short, or had an unusually slow pace, they were, almost without exception, related to drinking somehow. Clearly, the pattern was there: when it came to diet, exercise, and productivity . . . drinking was doing me no favors! In fact, it was getting to be a part of my lifestyle that more often than not, I considered to be a burden, and I increasingly contemplated how great it would be to just get out of my life. That's the tough part about drinking, though—even when we have clear evidence of why we shouldn't be doing it, if we still have the habitual impulse to drink, then all the logical reasons in the world don't add up to enough to pull the plug on it.

I did have some experience with giving up drinking for Lent every year and knew from those six weeks that it was a huge (albeit very temporary) upgrade to the overall quality of life. Even with those annual short-lived "proof of concept" experiments I always went back to drinking after Lent was over as I considered drinking a fairly fundamental part of my lifestyle, and frankly, it was tough to imagine actually making the leap to a life without it on a permanent basis.

Let's face facts: for centuries, alcohol has been a masterfully marketed product that has become deeply ingrained in our psyches as the primary catalyst for good times and the #1 tool for the job in making any social situation better. We are continuously bombarded through every possible media outlet that drinking is going to lead to good times, make us better looking, bring excitement and adventure, and, generally speaking, make our lives a whole lot more awesome. Everywhere we turn, drinking is glorified as our reward for hard work and the first thing to reach for to celebrate or socialize. It's so much a part of life in western world society that it's the only drug we have to explain why we are *not* taking in social situations. As an example, If you were at a party and someone was huffing airplane glue and offered you the paper bag to take a hit, you would not have to come up with an excuse as to why you were not going to partake! More than likely that sort of self-destructive activity would be done behind a closed door somewhere as whoever was doing it would on some level realize that's it some seriously deviant behavior that makes them look like a maniac (unless of course you specifically went to a glue huffing party, assuming such things exist).

Meanwhile, alcohol is a well-known killer toxin that is completely accepted and expected. The reality of that fact is pretty amazing. We have this drug, which the World Health Organization has classified as the leading cause of US mortality for ages 15-49, linked to 60 different diseases and a factor in over 3 million deaths globally each year. Not only that, but alcohol is a Class 1 carcinogen (the same classification as asbestos) tied to esophageal, liver, breast, head, and neck cancer, and even with these blazing neon warning lights, approximately 70% of people in the US still drink regularly. Alcohol is the third leading cause of preventable death each year in the US, and when it comes to deadly products expertly marketed, only tobacco has alcohol beat from an annual body count perspective. That said, a major difference with smoking is that it has a social stigma (sorry smokers!), which means that no excuses are necessary to not do it, and congratulations are offered to those who quit, unlike drinking, which pretty much seems to have a universal expectation of participation.

I point these things out not to rattle off statistics, as we all know that drinking is bad for us. We do it anyway because we enjoy how it makes us feel. I mention them in the context that I fully realize that a large mental obstacle that stands in the way of many people stopping their drinking is the anticipated dread of having to explain why they're not drinking. (We can probably all see the ridiculousness of having to justify the decision *not* to ingest a poisonous liquid, but that's the social world most of us are living in.)

So if this is something you can relate to, loving the idea of a life free of drinking but hating the thought of having to come up with reasons why you're not indulging, then BAR40 provides the perfect 52-week justification that truthfully explains the reason in a neat package. It's safe to say the "shock and awe" factor of you not drinking is largely dependent on how frequent of a drinker you are, of course. If you're someone who tends to always have a drink in hand in social settings, then it's fair to assume you will be asked the question of "where's your drink?" quicker and more frequently than someone who only occasionally imbibes. So if you, as I certainly was, are a card-carrying member of the drinking crowd, then those questions will definitely come up early and often. There's no getting around that eventuality, but you will see it's a conversation that you will very quickly lose any concern over.

When you're at your first dinner/party/work event/happy hour/wedding/holiday gathering (or the countless other scenarios that call for breaking out the booze), and the question pops up of, why you're not drinking the simple answer is some version of "I'm doing BAR40, it's a 52-week 'best year ever' challenge, based mainly on a fitness program and diet enhancements which cuts out added sugars and processed foods, and no alcohol is also part of it."

During the first year I did BAR40, I was traveling a lot for work, which seemed to always include a trade show, customer dinner, or social event where drinking was involved. Based on that, I can tell you from plenty of personal experience that this brief explanation will put an end to any worries you may have about explaining why you're not drinking. Probably the reason this explanation is so effective is because it reframes the conversation around this super impressive 52-week fitness program and shifts the focus away from drinking, which in reality is just one component of BAR40. Sure, it's a part of it but not the purpose. In reality, it just proves your hardcore commitment to dominating the next 52 weeks of your life in every possible area. You'll find that people are intrigued by and often envious of the fact that you're actually in the process of doing something they're going to do "someday": get back in shape and start working out. ("Someday" is called the 8th day of the week for good reason . . . it never arrives!)

Almost without exception, the response will be some version of the following or a combination:

Wow, a full year?!

That's awesome, good for you.

No way! Not even a few here and there? (Nope, I don't think there's a Junior Bar20 version!)

Whoa . . . that sounds cool, how's it going. Is it tough?

Very cool . . . I know who I'm calling to drive me around for the next year!

Wow, what are you going to do with all that money you're going to save?

Or some joke along the lines of . . . I quit drinking once, that was the toughest 15 minutes of my life!

The overwhelming reaction is an impressed curiosity, as I know you will soon see for yourself. One of the most surprising realizations I have had over the years of talking about BAR40 is just how many people quietly fantasize about stopping or cutting back on their drinking but have not locked in on the right opportunity or reason to do it. If it was a random conversation here or there, it wouldn't even be worth mentioning, but I have found it to be such a consistent theme with people steering the conversation toward questions about a non-drinking social life that only one conclusion can be drawn: there are a lot of people eager to talk with someone who is living an alcohol-free life and have a genuine curiosity about it. (Granted, many of these people may have a few in them already when you're having this conversation, of course, which may intensify their interest and enthusiasm for swearing off their own drinking, but plenty of these conversations will also take place before the drinks start flowing.)

In general, the growing "sober-curious" movement is proving to be a powerful force of change that is building momentum in dismantling this long-held social dogma that if you're not drinking you must be an alcoholic, a complete square and total bore, or in some way . . . just weird. All that seems to be changing, driven largely by the millennials who are "just not that into it" and are in part fueling this trend where being sober is a status symbol. As the expression goes, if you live long enough, you see it all! (Who would've thought the day would come when the coolest thing to do is not drink when you're 25 instead of wearing "Absolut Vodka" shirts!)

As always, when consumers show demand, the market will come up with the supply, and that is especially true with young affluent spenders in urban areas. "Mocktail" bars and dry nightclubs are becoming more common, and the fact that some top influencers on social sites like Instagram are beating the drum that "drinking is for old people" is moving the needle in big ways on how drinking is perceived.

Of course, once Hollywood stars get involved in something, that elevates the media attention to new levels. Brad Pitt, Bradley Cooper, Jada Pinkett Smith, Rob Lowe, Zac Efron, Ben Affleck, Blake Lively, John Stamos, Kendrick Lamar, Demi Lovato, Pharell Williams, Samuel Jackson, Jim Carrey, Tobey Maguire, and plenty more high profile celebrities have all made it well known that they want no part of drinking in their life and in doing so have played a part in normalizing the sober choice enough to the point where it's becoming a legitimate social shift in 2021. I spend time talking about this social pressure aspect of your not drinking because I know that it's something you are bound to encounter and I don't want any outside factors or peer pressure (perceived or actual) to take you off course. Also worth keeping in mind is that a big part of BAR40 means making the tough choices that serve long term goals for the best possible life and, frankly, that is an alien concept to the majority of people who do not have the discipline or commitment to personal accountability.

You will find that it does not take long to adopt the mindset of not being concerned with what anybody else is doing and be comfortable with the realization that the path you are on can be very different than those around you.

Last week I read a very interesting article related to this topic in the Harvard Business Review written by Michael Gervais, Ph.D. Gervais describes himself as a high-performance psychologist with clients that range from pro-athletes to Fortune 100 CEOs. This short article is titled "How to Stop Worrying What Other People Think of You" and provides a well written and concise overview of social anxiety and the ways it shows up in our life. Perhaps more importantly in the article is how we can mute those social alarm bells that we are all born with but often serve no purpose in our modern-day world.

To paraphrase a key point in the article: back in ancient days when our ancestors were out killing saber-toothed tigers for dinner, if they came back from the hunt empty-handed they faced the risk of being ostracized from the group for failing at their task. If that happened, they went hungry and probably cold as were likely to be boxed out of the nightly bonfire party. (Think Alec Baldwin in Glengarry Glenn Ross . . . "Fire is for closers!")

Social acceptance was literally a life or death scenario and as such, our evolutionarily development reflects that impulse to go along with the group and portray ourselves in a way that will be met with group approval. An easy example of this that all of us can relate to in one form or another is public speaking. Whether you're at a podium speaking to 500 people over a microphone or giving a monthly update to 20 people at a school committee meeting you have likely felt some change in your internal energy before speaking . . . a physical reaction to the anticipated moment of facing the crowd. Oftentimes this is felt as anxiety (stage fright jitters) or it can be a feeling of focused energy where you're adrenalized but ready. Personal feelings range across the spectrum from terrifying paralysis to a genuine excitement to get started but, at least in my many conversations ranging from novice to professional speakers, it seems no one is immune to some sort of physical reaction, even a slight one when it comes to speaking to a group. From an analytical and academic standpoint, this fear is completely irrational of course . . . there is absolutely nothing any of us should be anxious about in the simple act of speaking. It's not like we're being forced to jump out of a burning airplane or let tingan angry tarantula crawl up your arm, but we have an anticipatory physical reaction to public speaking that isn't much different than what we feel with physical danger. Just because it's a ridiculous phobia, that doesn't make it any less real . . . as we can attest to from our own experiences. For the record, I very much enjoy public speaking and welcome every opportunity to do it, but even after 25 years of frequent speaking I still get a fluttery feeling in my stomach a few minutes beforehand. I barely even notice it anymore and it's a subconscious physical reaction that I suspect will always occur. That said, the Zoom presentations of 2020 make for a different dynamic so that the normal sensation associated with public speaking can be lessened. (I did a virtual presentation last week in which there were 155 attendees and it may as well have been one person . . . it's a completely different psychological experience than presenting in-person and our physical reaction reflects the diminished "perceived threat"). I use this easy and relatable example of public speaking (often cited as people's #1 reported fear) to point out the power of our hardwired desire for "our pack" to accept us, and how this can work against us when we are attempting to do something that improves us as a person but is different than what others around us are doing.

Gervais refers to this limiting scenario as FOPO (fear of other people's opinion) and it's characterized by prioritizing (often obsessing) on how we look to others instead of what's most important for our own actual lives. Think about that for a second . . . we want so badly to "get likes" (both in social media and in daily in-person life) that we give other's opinions the final vote on how we live our own life. Fundamentally, it's easy to see that this pattern is not in alignment with any strategy we have to live our best life. On the positive side, this is a habit that we can overcome when we are conscious of it and make the mental effort to eliminate this undue emphasis on what others think. Even though this trait of seeking social acceptance is something we are programmed for, having awareness of its downsides, and practicing self-management to avoid them is a huge part of the solution.

To tie this into goals such as a 52-week sober challenge, one of the first and main steps is having clarity of purpose in what you are setting out to achieve and to making that your mission every day. (Gervais suggests creating a slogan that matches your personal philosophy and repeating it to yourself often) When you truly commit to that cause (whether it's not drinking or any challenge that involves doing the real work that most people around you are not willing to do) you become focused and driven to the point that any chatter from others about why it's too hard, can't happen, why bother?, do a cheat day, etc. just becomes background noise. It's not that you don't hear what these people are saying but rather if they are suggesting easier paths that are contrary to what you are seeking to accomplish, you can't help but find the conversation a waste of time. As your tolerance of time-wasting in your own life goes down you also may find yourself approaching zero-tolerance for conversations with other people trying to make a case for settling for easy mediocrity! Essentially your high-performance-oriented mind tends to drift back to more important topics of whatever you have on your day's to-do list in the pursuit of making it the best possible day. You start thinking in a higher frequency way and, trust me on this, you will start seeing people that can never seem to get anything done in their life as a whole different tribe than you. Once you start thinking at this higher level, the whole concept of feeling pressure to lower yourself down to their level for social acceptance feels ridiculous and you will simply stop caring. The process you will be going through in your pursuit of the next version of yourself is one of perseverance, grit, and daily determination, and this sort of growth mindset is how you process everything around you and the lens through which you see all decisions. That said, I have complete confidence in the fact that any worry or concern you may currently have about social pressure to have a drink will not last long and you will see it diminish every time you have an opportunity to build that muscle of mental toughness. As a personal example, I welcome any chance (although they are now few and far between) that someone will challenge me on why I'm not drinking in a social situation as it's always an interesting conversation to have with someone who is partially brainwashed and bloated from mindless consumerism in drinking a poison they've been sold believing it was going to make them successful, rich, and sexy. No mention of vomit in the bed, missing car keys, and 5:00am promises to never drink again found on any tequila billboards! While any feeling I may have had about wanting to fit in with that pack is long gone, I can still remember and empathize with those that are still in that mindset and I write about it because I know it's an important component in the whole process of taking a break from the booze.

On occasion, I still have people who ask if I mind if they drink around me. It's a polite question but still amusing in a way. To me, it's the equivalent of them unwrapping a few McDonald's Double Quarter Pounders and being concerned I'm going to be envious I don't have my own to enjoy. If I wanted to eat that food, there's nothing standing in my way of doing it except my decision to not have that sort of diet. It's the same with drinking. Unless you have some sort of medical condition or a court-ordered ankle monitor, there is nothing stopping me or you from drinking except for the choice not to. There isn't any feeling of sacrifice or missing out when you look at drinking from the perspective of what it's actually taking away from us rather than what people believe it to be adding for them.

Once you're on the path for a little while, you'll be settled in the saddle and the fact that you're not drinking will become expected and less of a conversation, especially with the people you see most often in your social life. For all of those people, the question tends to only come up the first time you're out with them and any time after that it just becomes something along the lines of How's the BAR40 going? question.

When you start experiencing life without drinking, you are going to be blown away by the changes, and again, the more you drink now, the more significant and profound the contrasts will be. If weight loss is one of your goals with BAR40, then get ready to love the results. If you start analyzing what's going on inside our body with relation to drinking and our weight, it's enough to make you wonder how anyone can ever hope to get into the shape they want to and still throw the drinks back. Doing both is a very steep uphill battle.

Here are five factors dealing with drinking and food that stack the deck against any weight loss effort:

- Alcohol is an appetite stimulant, so automatically when we're drinking we are inclined to eat more, and because alcohol also impairs judgment we tend to end up eating high calorie, low nutrition things like bar food, fast food and junk food instead of the healthier options we would normally choose when we're sober. For example, when's the last time you had a few drinks in you at 1:00 am and opted for a grilled chicken salad with dressing on the side?

- Alcohol acts as an anesthesia that basically disables the fuel gauge that tells us when we're full, so not only are we likely to be eating not the greatest food to begin with but, double whammy, we're much more likely to eat a lot more of it because we still feel hungry after the third slice of pizza.

- Because the body is unable to store alcohol as fat, it has to burn all those calories first before it can do anything with the food. So while our body is once again working overtime to get through all the drinks you poured down and basically process the poison out, the food you ate is being stored as fat until the alcohol is gone. Even if you're not drinking while you're eating, the alcohol contains excess sugars, which are also being stored as fat.

- Another point of note about what the body is doing with all those excess alcohol calories . . . it's basically converting them into heat, which is why we often get hot while we're drinking, but also increases blood flow to our face and neck. That extra blood causes our capillaries to dilate (and sometimes burst) leaving permanent souvenirs on your face in the form of broken blood vessels, especially on your cheeks and nose. Sort of like a visible hangover that's shouting . . . "stand back, big drinker coming through!"

- Not only is alcohol completely devoid of vitamins and minerals, it also acts as an inhibitor that blocks absorption of nutrients, specifically B1, B12, zinc and folic acid. The more often you drink, the more deficient you can become with those nutrients, and your body recognizes the shortage and sends out the "low level" alert in the form of hunger. So even if we have plenty of calories in us, we are still being prompted to eat, but the effort (and extra calories) do us no good because those nutrients won't be absorbed anyway.

- Last but not least, because drinking wreaks havoc on our sleep patterns, we tend to wake up the next day dragging our wagon and slightly exhausted. The body recognizes this low power level and reacts by saying, "get some more fuel on this fire!" and increases our appetite to boost our energy, which will be in excess of what our actual caloric need is. (Think of all the hung-over patrons in a diner any given Saturday morning, satisfying the craving for an omelet with home fries and bacon.) If drinking is a fairly frequent part of your life, then this pattern of being overly hungry the day after a big night is likely leading to a significant amount of overeating.

As mentioned in the earlier Sleep section, sleep deprivation is a fundamental factor in all sorts of problematic areas including disease, infection, obesity, and mood regulation, but we often tend to put it on the back burner of priorities. (If not a silent killer, then it's definitely a silent assaulter!) The topic of sleep and drinking is another area that you are going to see massive improvements with and may be something you don't even think about at the moment. Speaking from personal experience, I was definitely in this category in that generally, I felt what I considered to be fine the day after drinking. I refer to this as the "dirty windshield" syndrome because we don't realize just how obscured our visibility is until we clean the windshield and can once again see clearly. It wasn't until I stopped drinking that I realized that what I considered to be operating at full power was relative to the chronic poor sleep I was getting and not knowing what full potential strength was.

Another comparison you can make is using your work computer every day, which at some point picked up some sort of virus. It's not enough to prevent it from operating, and you can still get your work done on it, but you notice downloads are super slow or it takes a while to send emails with attachments, or maybe when you're trying to stream video it will always freeze up or the site will crash. Basically, just a bunch of small annoyances and, as such, you just deal it with every day and pretty much forget about it. Then, one weekend your company installs some new antivirus and debugging software, and you come in Monday morning to find your computer running at new lightning-fast speeds you never thought possible, and the differences across the board are amazing!

Within five minutes you will be asking yourself how you managed to use that thing for so long when it was running so slow. Of course, the answer is you didn't have this new 100% version to compare it with. This is the sort of performance boost that awaits when you cut out drinking, as you will soon see for yourself. Like other areas of improvement, the "before and after" differences will be proportionate to how much and how often you drink now and for how long you've been in that pattern. Even drinking small amounts of alcohol takes a toll on your sleep, so you will have noticeable improvements even if you are an infrequent drinker.

Think of how many times you have said or heard someone else say: "I'm not hung over, just tired." There are good reasons for this, and they run contrary to the common mentality of "a couple of drinks at night help me sleep." While partially true, alcohol is a depressant that will make you drowsy and help you fall asleep; that's where the good news ends when it comes to the rest of your night's sleep.

Clinical studies at multiple sleep labs using EEGs to measure subjects' brain wave activity overnight have found that one of the main reasons for sleep disruption is easily identified. Alpha brain waves begin occurring about halfway through the night, on average about five hours into sleep. Alpha waves are normally present during a state of calm wakefulness and combine with the delta waves (which occur during our deep sleep) to form an alpha-delta pattern that disrupts deep sleep from occurring. If you have ever gone to bed (passed out!) after drinking only to wake up in the middle of the night and have a tough time falling back asleep, this is likely one of the reasons. Basically, your circadian rhythm is thrown off by the chemical imbalance going on: alcohol comes in as a depressant, the brain releases a defense of stimulants to try to maintain a neutral balance . . . the alcohol eventually wears off, but the stimulants are still at work. These stimulants are sending the "time to wake up!" alert (and causing feelings of stress, anxiety, or generally unpleasant feelings) when the brain should be charging up its batteries and doing all the preventive brain maintenance that would have us waking up feeling rested and refreshed. Even if you do manage to sleep the whole night through, the damage to your sleep is being done in the sense that alcohol interrupts the three normal sleep patterns of light, deep, and REM from occurring. REM sleep is closely associated with mental restoration, cognitive processing, and mood regulation. When we fall asleep after drinking, we fall into a deep sleep and the first REM cycle that normally begins about 90 minutes into sleeping is blocked . . . sort of like we are under anesthesia. During this alcohol-induced deep sleep (let's call this the first half of your night), the body is metabolizing the alcohol and the excess sleep producing chemical (adenosine) out, which moves you into a light sleep pattern which can have frequent "micro-awakenings." You may not even be aware of these small disruptions that are preventing the true restorative benefits of sleep from taking place. If you have a Fitbit or any fitness device or app that provides you with a sleep report in the morning, you may be familiar with what the sleep pattern looks like in chart form, or there are plenty of examples in Google Images.

In addition, drinking disrupts sleep in the obvious ways that don't involve brain waves such as waking up because you're dehydrated and also the old standby . . . having to get up to use the bathroom. Any one of us can have a bad night's sleep once in a while and deal with it the next day; it may not be the best day ever, but we'll get through it. Generally, we can bounce back fairly quickly from an isolated event, but when drinking during the week is a fairly regular occurrence, then the accumulated effects over time stack up. This is the sort of incrementally building sleep deprivation that easily sneaks up on us and becomes a habitual sleep pattern. Here's a scenario to consider that you may be able to relate to: a few (or more) drinks are had in the evening, followed by a night of sleep that is missing critical sleep pattern components, get up feeling a little groggy but no big deal, go about your day gradually managing to shake off the cobwebs with the help of a couple cups of coffee and repeat the cycle later or tomorrow. If you drink currently, then having some version of this pattern is very common, considering the fact that even a couple glasses of wine two or three nights a week creates this accumulated deficit of sleep patterns that are missing the truly restful phases.

These are the aspects that I'm referring to in the example of the dirty windshield or computer running with a virus. When we're drinking alcohol at any sort of frequency (which statistically most social drinkers will report doing at least two to three days a week) the results are you end up continuously operating at diminished mental and physical levels without necessarily being aware of it.

Personally speaking, I was no stranger to having a few beers (or more!) any given night of the week, and if I had to take a health survey on how I felt any random morning, I would have put it at a 9 out of 10 most times. In looking back on it, the reality was that feeling is relative to the limitation of what we consider our best because of our chronic exhaustion.

I used to joke that my superpower was being able to fall asleep anywhere and anytime, as if I'd developed a skill that optimized energy efficiency and allowed me to "power down" at will. While it's true that if I put my head back, I could be asleep in less than a minute, most times I see it now as more just low-grade fatigue that was as constant as my sleep deprivation.

It's easy to go with the approach of "give me one good night's sleep and I'm all caught up," but in actuality, that's more a widely believed myth than the way it really works. Harvard Medical School did a study on chronic sleep deprivation that showed even sleeping an extra ten hours to compensate for two weeks' worth of being shortchanged just a small amount of sleep per night did not restore mental functioning and physical performance back to levels prior to the missed sleep. The study showed reaction times and ability to focus were actually worse than if the participants went a full night with no sleep instead of prolonged "short sleep." Based on the findings that even a short length of time with a slight loss of sleep has a significant impact on how we function during the day, just imagine what a lifestyle of disrupted sleep due to alcohol wreaking havoc on our sleep patterns amounts to! Living with chronically poor sleep also takes a big toll on our fitness goals. Anyone who regularly exercises knows that even when fully rested, some days the motivation to get your workout in can be tougher to muster up than others. When you add in the fact that you're fighting off a hangover, or just being tired, that workout becomes very tempting to skip altogether or get watered down by going through the motions to just get through it for a shorter amount of time at lessened intensity.

Last but not least on the subject of sleep and eliminating alcohol is the overall enhancement to mood and general emotional well-being. Any one of us can relate to the feeling of impatience or irritability we may have after a night of not enough sleep, but that's just the tip of the iceberg when it comes to the role sleep plays in regulating our emotional control panel. Sleep disruptions are directly linked to the majority of psychiatric and neurological mood disorders, so there are plenty of papers you can find online that provide detailed findings on the research. One interesting summary report is called "Overnight Therapy: The Role of Sleep in

Emotional Brain Processing" and is on the National Institute of Health site. It's a very interesting, very long, technical report with plenty of brain scan images, and it's definitely worth checking out if you're interested in learning more about this mysterious but critical function of sleep. A brief takeaway as it relates to BAR40: "Sleep loss was shown to amplify negative emotional consequences of disruptive daytime experiences while blunting the positive benefit associated with rewarding or goal-enhancing activities." In other words, losing out on sleep wires your brain to see the bad parts of your day as worse and the great parts as just okay.

REM sleep has a mission-critical job to do in making sure we are thinking and feeling our best every day and when we disable it by drinking (even those couple of drinks) there is a price to pay whether we think about it or not. This sort of emotional sabotage, in small or large degrees, is going on behind the scenes when you're operating continuously at half power, and you are very likely not even aware of it. When it comes to drinking versus not-drinking, this is an area, personally speaking, where I simply didn't know what I didn't know. Similar to the aspect of believing I felt physically great every day but realizing there was a whole different level to that after drinking was cut out, the mood and emotional side goes along the same path. In general, I tend to be a high-energy, positive person, but it wasn't until I was completely free of drinking for a few weeks that it fully dawned on me there was a whole higher gear of general positivity and passion for each day that I wasn't even aware of when I was chronically sleep-deprived. At the start of this Drinking section, I pointed out my intent to provide information on the advantages that cutting out drinking has for realizing the potential for your best year ever—hopefully, that was accomplished. Once again, I have nothing against drinking, and I have plenty of great friends and family who enjoy indulging. To each their own and if you're happy, then I'm happy, but I do want to create awareness about the reasons drinking takes away a lot more from our lives than it gives us.

My objective in the previous pages is to point out some of the very real advantages you will provide yourself by taking a break from drinking for the next 52 weeks. If after the year is done, you find that you miss it and want to go back to it, then so be it, but there's nothing to lose and only upside to be gained by sticking with the 52-week "challenge." If nothing else, you would have tried something new, done your overall health a huge favor, lost weight, improved your sleep, gotten in great shape, and saved thousands of dollars on alcohol in the process!

Depending on your current outlook on drinking, you may find yourself not going back to it at the end of the 52 weeks with the new realization, or perhaps confirmation of what you already suspected, that you find life in general is simply much better without alcohol in it. It really can be as simple as that. When you get right down to it, we all have some level of awareness that drinking is bad for us. Maybe we don't fully realize the extent and the various areas it impacts in our overall physical and emotional well-being but, on some level, we know it's not good for us. We choose to do it anyway for basically one reason . . . we enjoy the mood-altering effect it brings. That's it, that's the reason we do it. We tolerate all the negative aspects of drinking and its aftereffects to have the one benefit of liking the emotional state it brings. If the time comes when we stop enjoying it, then we have literally lost our only reason for drinking. If that occurs, the choice to delete it from your life becomes very simple. The pro/con list of drinking basically has a lot of minus marks and one plus, so when that goes away, it's pretty much a slam dunk case of getting rid of it. If quitting drinking permanently is one of your goals in doing BAR40, then this 52-week period is a perfect way to start the journey toward a life of sobriety and I strongly recommend reading some of the many books that are out there that go into detail about how alcohol actually works in our body and the brain chemistry changes that take place.

Seeing "how the sausage is made" as the expression goes helps provide a look behind the curtain and provides insight that can't be unseen. Once the power of alcohol is demystified and you read more about how the whole cycle works, it's actually somewhat difficult to find the idea of drinking to be appealing anymore. I had a high level of curiosity in drinking as it was a frequent part of my life for years and decided to do a "deep dive" in learning more about the whole subject of its effects and, in general, the hold it has on us as a society.

I would equate the learning experience to what I imagine it would be like if a die-hard steak lover spent a month working in a cattle slaughterhouse. I don't think it would be easy to go back to enjoying a big juicy porterhouse the same way after seeing first-hand how it came to arrive sizzling on your plate.

For anyone struggling to overcome alcohol addiction and wrestling with some variation of a "one day at a time" approach, I hope that they somehow find their way to coming at it from the approach of learning more about it to eliminate their actual desire to drink. Wanting to drink every day and struggling not to is an effort of prolonged willpower that data shows us leads to a high percentage of relapse. Alternatively, when the interest in drinking is eliminated, there is no mental struggle as it's simply a choice that has been made to remove it from your life. Once again, though, everyone has their own relationship with drinking ranging from "take it or leave it" to wishing they could stop but finding it difficult. My take on it is, "When the student is ready, the teacher appears" and if you find yourself ready to permanently stop drinking, reading *Alcohol Explained* which is on the BAR40 Suggested Reading List is going to be a big step in the direction of swearing off the booze. But be warned, you will not likely think about the "joy of drinking" the same way again!

Even if your plan is only to stop for the 52 weeks and then go back to normal drinking, *Alcohol Explained* will help reinforce the benefits of what you're doing and help eliminate any feelings of FOMO (fear of missing out) you may have around your drinking friends over the next year. I can easily remember my first year of doing BAR40. One of the questions I would get asked fairly often at social events was, "Don't you miss it?" The simple answer to that was yes, at first, I definitely missed the routine of it. After all, I had been a regular beer drinker for 20-plus years, so the act of not drinking was a pretty radical change! I was fully committed to the plan and never wavered during that year with having even one and I can tell you with certainty that, at least for me, after the first month or so it just becomes routine.

My plan was to do the 52 weeks and go back to drinking, which I did, but only to find that if I was somewhat sick of drinking before I stopped for the year, going back to it after the year was definitely a letdown. The one-year break was an amazing experience in all sorts of positive ways, and it cemented the realization that a sober life was, for me, better in every category . . . there's no simpler way to put it. I know that sounds absolutely crazy to you now if you're a regular drinker, so you will have to take my word for it until you start to experience it for yourself.

After going back to drinking and having a solid year of sober life experience to compare it to, the desire to drink was gone, and I decided to take it out of my life for the long term. So to fast forward to present day 2020, people still ask me if I miss it, and the answer is a definitive no. I have tons of great memories (and plenty of less than great ones of course!), and drinking can evoke feelings of nostalgia in the moments that in previous years would have been the textbook ideal day for throwing back some beers . . . hanging around the pool on a Saturday afternoon with friends, for example. I would compare it to watching *Fast Times at Ridgemont High* or *Dazed and Confused* . . . fun movies that can bring back fond memories of high school but after watching them, I don't have any desire to be back in the 10th grade. I look at drinking in a similar way, lots of fun memories of a time gone by that I have no interest in repeating. If there comes a time in the future where I once again decide that I would like to return to drinking, then certainly, nothing is stopping me. The simple fact of the matter is that I have come to enjoy feeling great every day with maximum productivity and energy more than I enjoyed drinking, and that realization makes eliminating it an easy decision.

I'll wrap up with the parting observation based on my own

experience doing BAR40 the first time: during the year, you will have urges and temptations to drink. That's completely normal as your brain is doing what it has been programmed to do, respond to triggers, and send the command to act accordingly. Just like if you're a passenger in a car and vehicle in front of you jams on the brakes . . . you automatically try to hit the brake pedal which doesn't exist on your side of the car . . . not because you consciously thought about it but because our subconscious knows what it's been programmed to do and is getting the job done before that sensory input reaches the logical decision making part of our brain.

As mentioned earlier in the Mindset-EQ section, our limbic system is the first stop for these sensory impulses, and it goes the same for drinking. Over time and repetition, we have written our own "if-then" programming codes. "If we are at a bar, concert, wedding, fishing trip . . . then drink." The details don't matter, but whatever activity you would normally have a drink doing, over time your subconscious has been conditioned to form the association so the next time you do it, of course, it will run the command to proceed as it has always done. Any of those associations are simply triggers, subconscious reactions by that highly efficient supercomputer brain of yours, and over time, those involuntary impulses will be replaced with the new subconscious program that does not include having a drink. Unless you are proactively avoiding those places and situations that you know will result in being a trigger, they are involuntary and unavoidable until they dissipate. A trigger is simply the alert to your conscious brain to perform some action, which is the craving . . . like seeing an orange juice commercial and having the urge to go to the kitchen for a tall glass of OJ. Cravings are a conscious function and one which you can simply override, which is the good news. Recognize a craving to drink for what it is, the quick process of an obsolete program being run that is no longer necessary, and in the process of being deleted.

William Porter, author of Alcohol Explained covers cravings at length in his writings as they are such a universal problem that lead to the undoing of so many well-intentioned sobriety plans. Oftentimes shedding light on the process of what's happening in our brain, both consciously and subconsciously, can be a huge help in dealing with the situation. A similar analogy would be when my daughter was younger and convinced there was a giant evil squirrel hiding in her closet in the middle of the night. I could certainly tell her that there was in fact no human-sized squirrel lurking behind the door but that would be a useless exercise. Instead, the lights had to come on, the closet door opened, and clothes moved to show that the closet was in fact clear. Only then would peaceful sleep be found again. Obviously, that's a simple solution to a simple problem but to the person fearing the squirrel or feeling the craving . . . the problem at that moment is as real as it gets!

So, to open the closet door and turn the lights on the craving problem let's dissect it using William Porter's 4-phase model. First, there is the fantasizing part. In our heads, we are thinking about how great it would be to have a drink (or 5). We make this out to be a much more fulfilling event in our heads than it actually is of course . . . that's our brain playing a drinking highlight reel that the liquor industry can only hope to someday replicate in its effectiveness at convincing you to drink! This fantasizing is a form of slow torture in that we keep thinking about the object of our desire (this can just as easily be food or anything we are trying to gain some better control over but for this example let's just stick to alcohol).

The fantasizing is certainly distracting but not a huge problem in itself. The next phase of craving is when it starts to become a slippery slope, though . . . this is the stage where you start to entertain the idea that maybe just one drink wouldn't be a big deal. If you were to freeze the scene in the movie at this moment . . . this is where the trouble begins. While we are escalating our fantasy to the realm of "maybe . . . just maybe" status we are now in the high-risk area for phase #3.

This is the phase where there is a real risk of "falling off the wagon" as the expression goes because it's at this point that the subconscious shows up on the scene to take control of the situation. One of the amazing superpowers this brain of ours has is the ability to become very efficient at task management and decision making and while most of the time that can work in our favor at executing tasks without much thought, it can also work against us . . . like in this scenario. The subconscious recognizes that in our conscious brain we are wasting a lot of brainpower with the thinking of, just one, I'll quit tomorrow, it's been a tough week, I deserve to relax, it would be great to try this new wine, etc. and it identifies that it needs to step in to put this nonsense to rest and makes the decision for you that you will, in fact, have a drink. Problem solved, says the ruthlessly efficient subconscious . . . decision made and onto the next thing on the list.

Now back to our conscious brain for the final stage of

craving (at which point your resolve to not drink is really in "red alert" status) which is basically when we are mentally scrolling through our standard "go-to" excuses and rationalization playbook looking for one to latch on to that will allow you come to some form of peace with the idea that you are in fact about to do what you earlier in the day were committed not to do.

That is a summary of the life cycle of craving and I hope it helps show just how much control we have over this situation, to begin with.

Fundamentally, the whole thing need not progress past the first phase of fantasizing. If you think about it, there isn't really harm in that tendency and it would be difficult to turn off even if we wanted to . . . Our natural tendency is to have fantasies all the time about the whole range of topics in our life. We fantasize about winning the lottery, but it stops there. For most of us, simply thinking about winning the $300 million Powerball doesn't lead to us drain our bank accounts to buy tickets and quit our jobs in expectation of winning. It's just a harmless fantasy that does not lead to any action.

With drinking, it's a simple (but not always as easy) mental step where we fully commit to the idea that we are not drinking, there is simply no other alternative. This small but mighty step ensures that like the lottery example, there is not going to be any fantasy to action conversion. This "burn the boats" mentality that alcohol will not be had for the next 52 weeks is an airtight capsule that will not allow Stages 2, 3, and 4 to enter into the equation. A similar example can be found with expecting mothers all the time. There are always exceptions of course, but statistically speaking women who are pregnant are in the mindset that drinking is off the table for the next nine months or so. In a lot of cases, the mom-to-be is very vocal in expressing her impatience to "get this margarita party started as soon as this baby is born" but this is just harmless fantasizing as they know deep down that they will not be having that margarita party while they're expecting.

I can't emphasize this enough: if you seal the deal in your mind that you will not be drinking for the next year and do not leave the door open even a crack with "cheat days" and "special occasions,'" then daily life becomes infinitely easier in that you'll likely be thinking about drinking . . . we are surrounded by drinking reminders every day as it's all around us . . . but you will not be at any risk of actually doing it because you have mentally eliminated the possibility. Your subconscious will never even be involved because there is no decision you are grappling with. The decision is made and does not even need to be considered for the next 52 weeks and at that point, you can re-evaluate whether or not you want to re-introduce drinking into your life. I think you will be absolutely amazed at the game-changing mental transformation you have when you 100% commit to yourself that alcohol will not be entering your body for the next 52 weeks. End of story. Or as my friends in the UK say . . . done and dusted.

Keeping that in mind and recognizing the process at work makes sticking to your 52-week sober plan just one more daily success to add to your journal and one more opportunity to build that mental toughness!

One final note on drinking as I write this on November 22nd, 2020. Covid-19 has been life-changing for all of us in every way imaginable (and some unimaginable) and one of the unfortunate trend developments has been the significant uptick in alcohol consumption. For some people, that means the drinking habit they had going into Covid has swelled into a full-grown problem now that they don't have the guardrails and structure that their normal 8-5 office routine provided. For other people, it may mean that their once a month glass of wine at dinner has turned into Zoom happy hours three times a week and they've found that when the Zoom call is over at 6:00 pm they tend to keep drinking the rest of the night. For others, the change in schedule and not going into their office has meant that instead of having their first drink of the day at 6:00 pm it has crept up into the afternoon, and now eight months into this new world order, their drinking is tracking toward the "it's noon somewhere" philosophy. Alcohol is an addictive substance, and like any other addictive substance . . . the more we do it, the more we tend to do.

One study conducted in August 2020 by the American Addiction Center (AAC) asked 3000 participants about their drinking at home during Covid: 36% of men and 26% of women surveyed reported drinking while on the job. There was not a corresponding question asking if those same people were typically drinking in normal times while they were at their actual place of work but, let's face it, most of them probably were not.

In a lot of ways, 2020 has proved to be the perfect cocktail recipe (as it were) for a drinking problem to develop. Ingredient #1 is social isolation, stress, anxiety, depression, and other mental ailments that have been worsened by the 24/7 onslaught of Covid news and worry. Ingredient #2 is a general normalizing of excess drinking and afternoon

Quarantini parties rationalized with the reasoning that, Hey, it's the end of the world . . . bottoms up! Finally, add in the fact that many people are now working from home and are operating in an environment without direct interaction with co-workers and managers and are able to freely drink without any concerns of "getting caught." Can't smell the booze on Zoom, right!? (I've heard that on more than one call.) Statistics on retail alcohol sales (beer, wine, and liquor) showed a huge year-over-year jump starting in March but that's not any real surprise considering restaurant and bar closures coupled with people stockpiling in the event of a supply shortage. A more telling indicator of the increased drinking trend are treatment facilities around the country reporting a surge in both inquiries and new patients seeking help for alcohol use disorders. Data shows that the areas hardest hit by Covid often have a correspondingly high rate of increase in patients seeking addiction treatment, which isn't surprising considering the well-established connection between drinking and stress-management attempts.

From my perspective, I don't need the statistics to tell the tale . . . simply having conversations with people of various generations in all different walks of life make it clear that many of us or our loved ones are doing a lot more imbibing in this pandemic world and it's not always going so well. I have a somewhat unique vantage point in that the BAR40 program is becoming well known, along with its 52-week sober challenge. Based on that I often find myself in conversations with people that are specifically interested in talking about drinking . . . or more to the point . . . not drinking!

It's validating to know that BAR40 is helping people manage

this part of their lives and providing the motivation and reason to set their sights on the best year ever including stopping a drinking habit before it really sneaks up and bites you. This pandemic reality is tough enough without adding in the extra set of life-blasting consequences that a drinking problem can reign down on you and your loved ones that are on your "quaran-team."

I'll wrap up this section by simply saying that if you feel like your drinking is starting to get a little bit out of hand then it almost certainly is. I encourage anyone reading this to take the 52-week sober challenge for all the reasons I wrote about earlier, but if you find yourself in the category of "growing concerned" (or the people around you are pointing out your drinking is concerning to them) then I emphatically suggest you give yourself a break from the booze. If you decide after the year is done you miss drinking and want to get back to it then knock yourself out, it will be right there waiting for you like a book you put down on the coffee table with the page saved. In the world of uncertainty we live in, one constant that you can count on is that whatever drinking habits you have now will be right there waiting for you if you decide to drink again. The good news is that in your year-long break you will look and feel your best, have a truly restful sleep, save money, and have a huge mental boost with regard to clarity and energy. Finally, alcohol wreaks havoc on your immune system so if your aim is to stay Covid-free, avoiding alcohol is definitely a solid play in keeping your biological shields at full power.

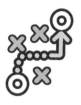

Getting Started

N ow that we've covered the fundamentals, the time has almost arrived to get this BAR40 ball rolling! First, a few notes on next steps to take now that you've had a chance to read the various sections.

Choose your official BAR40 start date — This will be the day when the 52-week/365-day journey begins. If you're ready to start today, then by all means, go for it, but more than likely you will prefer to spend some time on the pre-planning for your goals, diet plan and fitness objectives/workout schedule. Also, if you're looking to get some last drinks in before your one-year (or longer!) hiatus from alcohol begins, then this scheduled start date provides a runway for that as well.

Give some serious consideration to what your main goals are going to be for this coming year — These goals are fundamental to what you consider to be the most valuable pursuits to reach the best version of yourself. Envision your future self one year from now having just completed BAR40 and imagine what you would be most proud of achieving . . . what would make you look back and say, I finally did it! What accomplishments or wish list items are on your life's to-do list but for whatever reason you have not checked them off yet. Think about any of the times you have said, Someday I'm going to _____, and fill in the blank. Let this year be the "someday" that you have been referring to all this time. If you're having a hard time deciding or coming up with the goals, then by all means, have a conversation with someone close to you who may have immediate insight on a target area of your life that is eluding you at the moment. The only word of caution I would give in that area is not agreeing to anyone else's idea of a goal unless it truly resonates as something of the highest personal importance to you. These goals will be a big part of your motivation over the next 52 weeks and if you're not highly invested in them for yourself, they may prove difficult to stick with.

Put together a fitness plan — Depending on your lifestyle now and whether exercise is already a part of it, this could be an area that you need to build from the ground up. On the other hand, you may already have activities you regularly do and plan on dialing up the frequency, mileage, or intensity and adding some additional components to it. Wherever you currently are in your life with an exercise routine (even if there isn't one at the moment!) it's worthwhile to put some thought into what part of the day you will be setting aside for your workout. I realize that life is busy, the days can be hectic, and schedules can change week to week. This is exactly why it's important to invest some time on determining what time of day is going to be most compatible with your schedule based on the existing work, family, or other assorted commitments we all have.

If you plan on spending approximately one hour per day, five days a week exercising, then that provides a clear specific block of time to enter into your week's schedule at the appropriate time that works best for you. The expression "a goal without a plan is just a wish" is definitely applicable here. Taking the approach of figuring it out day by day or getting to it when everything else on the day's to-do list is done can be a recipe for a lot of missed workouts.

One suggestion is to try looking at that workout time like work meetings, doctor's appointments, or anything that you normally would not cancel unless you absolutely had to. These are basically important meetings with yourself, and if it helps, enter them into whatever calendar app you use and consider them to be the firm commitments that they are.

I know it can be tough to plan too far out sometimes, but perhaps at some point every weekend when you're looking at the coming week's schedule you make sure that however many days you plan on exercising have a pre-determined spot. This step of scheduling them is a highly effective commitment device and is much more consistent than making your workout an afterthought that needs to be squeezed in every day.

Having run many midnight miles over the years (because skipping a workout after I lost track of time is not an option I accept) I can tell you from ample experience that having a planned schedule in place is a much easier way to go about it and something you will thank yourself for!

Plan your diet modifications — This is as simple as making a list of what you're normally eating now (breakfast, lunch, dinner, and snacks) and next to those items noting what the better substitutes are going to be. Some of the foods will have obvious better alternatives and for anything you're not sure on, the Food Target that's included in the earlier Diet section will be a huge help for immediate reference, or you can download the PDF from the *On Target Living* site or order one from their site. You can also use the time before your scheduled BAR40 start day to keep a food journal, as they can be very helpful in putting together an accurate and complete record of what a normal day entails as opposed to trying to list everything from memory. I think you'll find the whole substitution and improvement mindset to be one that you come to take a lot of satisfaction in over the next year. Like other habits toward the "best you" that you will be building up in the coming year, there is definitely an addictive factor in continuously finding new ways to ratchet your diet up a notch. It's similar to the feeling of cleaning out a neglected drawer or closet and loving the new extra space. This can quickly transition to the urge to find some other space to declutter and that's how you may find yourself thinking about what you eat and drink. When we get a new hammer, all we see are nails!

No question about it, your shopping list will look different and much healthier. I know the ultimate goal is improved health and it goes without saying that cutting down on saturated fats and processed food offers significant benefits even if you can't necessarily see them. In addition, though, there will be noticeable differences when you start "burning cleaner fuel" in that your energy will increase, mental clarity sharpens, and you will in general just feel better overall. Add the fact that you will be losing some weight in the meantime and it's a win on top of a win!

If one of your main goals is in fact losing weight, just keep in mind that it's not an overnight process (just like the pounds were not accumulated overnight) but stick with it and the results will happen. There is a spot in the journal for your weekly weight, so I encourage you to use that for a weekly check in. The scale is not the be all and end all fitness measuring device obviously and as we work out more, we are improving our physique but also adding muscle which skews the numbers in the sense that you may be adding muscle weight but losing fat pounds. No matter what, if weight loss is your goal, one of the things that the $930 million dollars has proven is that the weekly trip to the scale increases your personal accountability and helps regulate your eating choices during the rest of the week.

Suggested Reading List — As I have mentioned throughout the book, there is a tremendous amount of information that has been published about each of the main topics of this book: personal excellence, fitness, diet, goal setting, mindfulness, and drinking. What I believe to be the unique aspect of BAR40 is the approach toward enhancing each of these areas simultaneously with the reasoning that each part of our life is interconnected although often it's not proactively looked at in that way.

For instance, I'm sure you can think of people in your life that are in great physical shape but who are monsters to be around from a personality perspective. Or... other people who have a great outlook on life and a joy to be around but are in terrible physical condition. There are all sorts of variables and moving parts in our lives and it's a tall order to get everything dialed in, but the biggest challenge can be just finding the start of the path to begin the journey. This is where BAR40 comes in to help. One analogy could be from a construction perspective. My book is designed to help provide the tools and blueprint for you to build your dreamhouse of the ultimate you. Only you can do the actual labor and put in the work to get the construction done but having a plan to work from helps ensure the end results are exactly what you've always wanted.

So much of everything in this book comes down to creating a mindset and life philosophy of forward motion and personal growth through constant improvement. This is not a "power of positive thinking . . . just believe good things will happen and stand by for the magic results to appear" approach. It's developing the habit of personal accountability and perseverance through repeated choices every day. Often this means doing what others aren't willing to do, whether it be forgoing dessert, getting that workout in when you're tired, or bypassing the booze.

Your process will involve constantly elevating yourself to the next level in work, life, and health. When these various gears are meshing together you are going to have this rising tide effect of improvements throughout your life paying huge dividends to not only you but all those around you in your work and your personal life.

One of the main benefits that BAR40 provides is this condensed library of books that are on the Suggested Reading List. As mentioned earlier, there is an ocean of information out there and finding the most useful resources is a daunting and time-consuming endeavor. My objective here is eliminating your need for a lot of frustrating trial and error and providing you with a distilled "best in class" selection of what I consider very useful books in close alignment with the BAR40 objectives. Each one of these authors has done an excellent job in covering their respective topics clearly and with expertise and trying to provide watered down snippets of their books here would be a disservice to you.

BAR40 is a self-guided journey that calls for you to identify the target improvement areas in your life and execute those changes. It's as simple but not as easy as that: identify, adapt and evolve, and I think these books will provide you significant help along the way. I have included 13 books on the Suggested Reading List, basically spacing them out so it's a new book selection every four weeks; the summary of each appears in the journal at the designated week. You may be thinking . . . Whoa, hang on a second buddy . . . you're saying I have to find time to read an extra book a month now!? (I know that may have flashed across your mind.) To that, I would look at it like this: almost all of the books are under 300 pages, which means that if you simply read ten pages per day, then you will easily be finishing these books each month before starting on the next one. I'll even go so far as to say you're going to be enjoying them so much that you'll be burning through them and looking forward to diving into the next one!

Audio books are always an option as well if you'd rather listen than read; my preference happens to be the paper version as I tend to retain it better and can easily go back to re-read any key areas, but of course that choice is yours.

As far as cost goes, all of these books are available as used options on Amazon or eBay if you prefer that over buying new ones and they may also be available from your local library in paper, e-book, or audio versions. Also, consider the amount of money that BAR40 is putting back into your pocket in the form of savings on alcohol which will likely far exceed the cost of the Suggested Reading List. A conservative estimate of social weekend drinkers put the annual cost of drinking at about $2,000 and if you drink during the week as well, then your annual financial could easily be a lot more. Google "annual alcohol spending calculator" and you will find some sites that pop up which will quickly give you your weekly, monthly, and annual spending when you plug in some (honest!) answers about your normal weekly drinking.

On a closing note, my sincere hope is that you find the BAR40 program as life changing as I believe it can be for you. Every aspect of this book comes from my personal experience and approaches which continue to be highly effective in living the best year ever, every year.

Let this journal be your daily training partner not just for diet and exercise purposes but also for the larger topics of daily success and areas for growth. Review your progress and write reminders and notes to yourself weeks or months ahead. Put this journal to full use every day and let it bring out the full potential in you . . . it should be a tattered wreck from handling after a full year of daily use!

My prediction is that the practices you will develop will make this commitment to personal excellence the operating system your life runs on and each subsequent year will be even better than the one before it. Please feel free to email me anytime at eric@bar40.org and let me know how you're doing. Here's wishing you the best year ever!

Stay safe and be well,

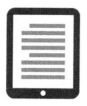

Suggested Reading List

Week 1   *The Power of Habit* by Charles Duhigg

Week 5   *You Are Your Own Gym* by Mark Lauren

Week 9   *On Target Living* by Chris Johnson

Week 13 *Emotional Intelligence 2.0*
by Travis Bradberry and Jean Greaves

Week 17 *Incognito* by David Eagleman

Week 21 *Why We Sleep* by Matthew Walker

Week 25 *Getting Things Done* by David Allen

Week 29 *How to Win Friends and Influence People*
by Dale Carnegie

Week 33 *The Way of the Seal* by Mark Divine

Week 37 *How Emotions Are Made* by Lisa Feldman Barrett

Week 41 *The 7 Habits of Highly Effective People*
by Stephen R. Covey

Week 45 *The Slight Edge* by Jeff Olson

Week 49 *Alcohol Explained* by William Porter

Using the Journal

You may have heard the expression, "Responsibility is ownership of activities, but accountability is ownership of results." This journal is designed to be your daily tool for optimal personal accountability. You are starting on a 52-week mission that is highly results-oriented. Specifically, achieving the goals you have identified as priorities and adopting a lifestyle that will, over the course of the next 12 months, help you maximize your potential in all areas of your life. This journal is set up for daily use and is much more inclusive than a standard fitness journal.

In keeping with the concept that the best year ever is built upon the bricks of many best days, the journal provides a space to reflect on memorable moments of each day, whether they be positive or negative. This simple act of putting pen to paper brings many proven benefits including organizing your thoughts, helping identify priorities, boosting creativity, and reducing stress. Taking the step of looking back on your day and writing about it will often shift your perspective and put situations in a new light which will influence your behavior and decisions going forward. Also included are "daily successes" which help create the habit throughout the day of being on the lookout for ways to do whatever it is you're doing in a slightly better way. (Not to mention, looking back at previous pages and seeing about 20 successes a week is a great way to keep "catching yourself doing something right"!)

Each day brings different tasks and requirements of your time, so there is a spot for "Today's Goals" that can be completed each morning or the night before and this helps prioritize your daily "must do" items in a simple and straightforward way.

At the end of each week there is a space to do a quick recap of the highlights of the week as well as set priorities for the next week.

As this is also a fitness journal, there is plenty of space each day to record your workout summary and any notes of interest, as well as anything you want to include regarding your diet. If weight loss is one of your intentions for the next year, then you will also find a space to include your weekly weight. (As mentioned in earlier pages, weight loss studies have shown conclusive data that a weekly weight check is in the habits of people that have not only lost weight but also kept it off over the years.) Last but not least, there is a "Reminder From Your Past Self" spot that can be used any time you want to do an exercise in time travel and send a message to your future self that will be read weeks or months down the road.

Remember that each of us is the author of our own life story based on our choices, habits and actions. At the same time . . . history is not destiny and each day gives us a fresh page to write on and decide where the plot goes next. Write the story that will make your future self proud.

Daily Journal Pages

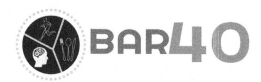

WEEK 1

Date: _____

MONDAY

Day in review - What made today memorable?

TUESDAY

Day in review - What made today memorable?

WEDNESDAY

Day in review - What made today memorable?

THURSDAY

Day in review - What made today memorable?

> "There are only two days in the year that nothing can be done. One is called yesterday and the other is called tomorrow, so today is the right day to love, believe, do, and mostly live." — *Dalai Lama*

Workout Summary & Diet Notes:	TODAY'S GOALS	DONE?
Sleep Hours **Daily Successes:** 1. 2. 3.	1. ____ 2. ____ 3. ____ 4. ____	○ ○ ○ ○

Workout Summary & Diet Notes:	TODAY'S GOALS	DONE?
Sleep Hours **Daily Successes:** 1. 2. 3.	1. ____ 2. ____ 3. ____ 4. ____	○ ○ ○ ○

Workout Summary & Diet Notes:	TODAY'S GOALS	DONE?
Sleep Hours **Daily Successes:** 1. 2. 3.	1. ____ 2. ____ 3. ____ 4. ____	○ ○ ○ ○

Workout Summary & Diet Notes:	TODAY'S GOALS	DONE?
Sleep Hours **Daily Successes:** 1. 2. 3.	1. ____ 2. ____ 3. ____ 4. ____	○ ○ ○ ○

FRIDAY

Day in review - What made today memorable?

SATURDAY

Day in review - What made today memorable?

SUNDAY

Day in review - What made today memorable?

Highlights of this Week

1.
2.
3.
4.
5.

Top Priorities For Next Week

1.   4.
2.   5.
3.   6.

Weekly Summary (good/bad/other/weight/etc.)

Reminder From Your Past Self

Workout Summary & Diet Notes:

Sleep Hours

Daily Successes:

1.
2.
3.

TODAY'S GOALS

DONE?

1.

2.

3.

4.

Workout Summary & Diet Notes:

Sleep Hours

Daily Successes:

1.
2.
3.

TODAY'S GOALS

DONE?

1.

2.

3.

4.

Workout Summary & Diet Notes:

Sleep Hours

Daily Successes:

1.
2.
3.

TODAY'S GOALS

DONE?

1.

2.

3.

4.

Fitness Highlights of this Week

1.
2.
3.
4.
5.

Weekly Fitness Notes

RHR

BP

Total Distance (in miles)

Week   Year

Weight

WEEK 1

The Power of Habit

I mentioned in the Introduction section that this was going to be first on the Suggested Reading List and the reason for that is the book does such a fantastic job of exploring how central a role habits play in our daily lives and how we can use this knowledge to harness the power of the subconscious. There's definitely a good amount of science based research in here that pulls back the curtain on how our brain works, but Duhigg delivers it in such an enjoyable way with plenty of anecdotes that it makes the book as entertaining as it is enlightening. It's basically a how-to manual for ending or creating habits and you may find yourself actively looking for more areas of your life to attack with your new skills. I almost decided to start smoking just to have a new habit to quit! Just kidding on that but you'll see what I mean . . . it's very fulfilling to develop this new tool set for managing your subconscious and kicking off BAR40 is a perfect time to apply what you'll learn.

WEEK 2

Date: _____

MONDAY
Day in review - What made today memorable?

TUESDAY
Day in review - What made today memorable?

WEDNESDAY
Day in review - What made today memorable?

THURSDAY
Day in review - What made today memorable?

"Time is what we want most, but what we use worst." — *William Penn*

Workout Summary & Diet Notes:	TODAY'S GOALS	DONE?
Sleep Hours	1. _____	◯
	2. _____	◯
Daily Successes:	3. _____	◯
1. _____	4. _____	◯
2. _____		
3. _____		

Workout Summary & Diet Notes:	TODAY'S GOALS	DONE?
Sleep Hours	1. _____	◯
	2. _____	◯
Daily Successes:	3. _____	◯
1. _____	4. _____	◯
2. _____		
3. _____		

Workout Summary & Diet Notes:	TODAY'S GOALS	DONE?
Sleep Hours	1. _____	◯
	2. _____	◯
Daily Successes:	3. _____	◯
1. _____	4. _____	◯
2. _____		
3. _____		

Workout Summary & Diet Notes:	TODAY'S GOALS	DONE?
Sleep Hours	1. _____	◯
	2. _____	◯
Daily Successes:	3. _____	◯
1. _____	4. _____	◯
2. _____		
3. _____		

FRIDAY

Day in review - What made today memorable?

SATURDAY

Day in review - What made today memorable?

SUNDAY

Day in review - What made today memorable?

Highlights of this Week

1. _____
2. _____
3. _____
4. _____
5. _____

Reminder From Your Past Self

Top Priorities For Next Week

1. _____ 4. _____
2. _____ 5. _____
3. _____ 6. _____

Weekly Summary (good/bad/other/weight/etc.)

Workout Summary & Diet Notes:	TODAY'S GOALS	DONE?
Sleep Hours	1.	○
	2.	○
Daily Successes:	3.	○
1.	4.	○
2.		
3.		

Workout Summary & Diet Notes:	TODAY'S GOALS	DONE?
Sleep Hours	1.	○
	2.	○
Daily Successes:	3.	○
1.	4.	○
2.		
3.		

Workout Summary & Diet Notes:	TODAY'S GOALS	DONE?
Sleep Hours	1.	○
	2.	○
Daily Successes:	3.	○
1.	4.	○
2.		
3.		

Fitness Highlights of this Week

1.
2.
3.
4.
5.

Weekly Fitness Notes

RHR

BP

Total Distance (in miles)		Weight	
Week	Year		**WEEK 2**

WEEK 3

Date: _____

MONDAY

Day in review - What made today memorable?

TUESDAY

Day in review - What made today memorable?

WEDNESDAY

Day in review - What made today memorable?

THURSDAY

Day in review - What made today memorable?

"Attract what you expect, reflect what you desire, become what you respect, mirror what you admire."

Workout Summary & Diet Notes:	TODAY'S GOALS	DONE?
Sleep Hours	1.	◯
	2.	◯
Daily Successes:	3.	◯
1.		
2.	4.	◯
3.		

Workout Summary & Diet Notes:	TODAY'S GOALS	DONE?
Sleep Hours	1.	◯
	2.	◯
Daily Successes:	3.	◯
1.		
2.	4.	◯
3.		

Workout Summary & Diet Notes:	TODAY'S GOALS	DONE?
Sleep Hours	1.	◯
	2.	◯
Daily Successes:	3.	◯
1.		
2.	4.	◯
3.		

Workout Summary & Diet Notes:	TODAY'S GOALS	DONE?
Sleep Hours	1.	◯
	2.	◯
Daily Successes:	3.	◯
1.		
2.	4.	◯
3.		

FRIDAY

Day in review - What made today memorable?

SATURDAY

Day in review - What made today memorable?

SUNDAY

Day in review - What made today memorable?

Highlights of this Week

1.
2.
3.
4.
5.

Reminder From Your Past Self

Top Priorities For Next Week

1.   4.
2.   5.
3.   6.

Weekly Summary (good/bad/other/weight/etc.)

Workout Summary & Diet Notes:

Sleep Hours

Daily Successes:

1.
2.
3.

TODAY'S GOALS

DONE?

1.

2.

3.

4.

○
○
○
○

Workout Summary & Diet Notes:

Sleep Hours

Daily Successes:

1.
2.
3.

TODAY'S GOALS

DONE?

1.

2.

3.

4.

○
○
○
○

Workout Summary & Diet Notes:

Sleep Hours

Daily Successes:

1.
2.
3.

TODAY'S GOALS

DONE?

1.

2.

3.

4.

○
○
○
○

Fitness Highlights of this Week

1.
2.
3.
4.
5.

Weekly Fitness Notes

RHR

BP

Total Distance
(in miles)

Week

Year

Weight

WEEK 3

WEEK 4

Date: _____

MONDAY
Day in review - What made today memorable?

TUESDAY
Day in review - What made today memorable?

WEDNESDAY
Day in review - What made today memorable?

THURSDAY
Day in review - What made today memorable?

> "If you do what you've always done, you'll get what you've always gotten."
> — *Tony Robbins*

Workout Summary & Diet Notes:	TODAY'S GOALS	DONE?
Sleep Hours	1. _____	○
	2. _____	○
Daily Successes:	3. _____	○
1. _____	4. _____	○
2. _____		
3. _____		

Workout Summary & Diet Notes:	TODAY'S GOALS	DONE?
Sleep Hours	1. _____	○
	2. _____	○
Daily Successes:	3. _____	○
1. _____	4. _____	○
2. _____		
3. _____		

Workout Summary & Diet Notes:	TODAY'S GOALS	DONE?
Sleep Hours	1. _____	○
	2. _____	○
Daily Successes:	3. _____	○
1. _____	4. _____	○
2. _____		
3. _____		

Workout Summary & Diet Notes:	TODAY'S GOALS	DONE?
Sleep Hours	1. _____	○
	2. _____	○
Daily Successes:	3. _____	○
1. _____	4. _____	○
2. _____		
3. _____		

FRIDAY

Day in review - What made today memorable?

SATURDAY

Day in review - What made today memorable?

SUNDAY

Day in review - What made today memorable?

Highlights of this Week

1.
2.
3.
4.
5.

Reminder From Your Past Self

Top Priorities For Next Week

1. 4.
2. 5.
3. 6.

Weekly Summary (good/bad/other/weight/etc.)

Workout Summary & Diet Notes:

Sleep Hours

Daily Successes:

1.
2.
3.

TODAY'S GOALS

1.
2.
3.
4.

DONE?

○
○
○
○

Workout Summary & Diet Notes:

Sleep Hours

Daily Successes:

1.
2.
3.

TODAY'S GOALS

1.
2.
3.
4.

DONE?

○
○
○
○

Workout Summary & Diet Notes:

Sleep Hours

Daily Successes:

1.
2.
3.

TODAY'S GOALS

1.
2.
3.
4.

DONE?

○
○
○
○

Fitness Highlights of this Week

1.
2.
3.
4.
5.

Weekly Fitness Notes

RHR

BP

Total Distance (in miles)

Week [ ] Year [ ]

Weight [ ]

WEEK 4

WEEK 5

Date: _____

MONDAY

Day in review - What made today memorable?

TUESDAY

Day in review - What made today memorable?

WEDNESDAY

Day in review - What made today memorable?

THURSDAY

Day in review - What made today memorable?

"Success is not final; failure is not fatal: It is the courage to continue that counts." — *Winston S. Churchill*

Workout Summary & Diet Notes:	TODAY'S GOALS	DONE?
Sleep Hours **Daily Successes:** 1. 2. 3.	1. _____ 2. _____ 3. _____ 4. _____	○ ○ ○ ○
Sleep Hours **Daily Successes:** 1. 2. 3.	1. _____ 2. _____ 3. _____ 4. _____	○ ○ ○ ○
Sleep Hours **Daily Successes:** 1. 2. 3.	1. _____ 2. _____ 3. _____ 4. _____	○ ○ ○ ○
Sleep Hours **Daily Successes:** 1. 2. 3.	1. _____ 2. _____ 3. _____ 4. _____	○ ○ ○ ○

FRIDAY

Day in review - What made today memorable?

SATURDAY

Day in review - What made today memorable?

SUNDAY

Day in review - What made today memorable?

Highlights of this Week

1. _____
2. _____
3. _____
4. _____
5. _____

Reminder From Your Past Self

Top Priorities For Next Week

1. _____ 4. _____
2. _____ 5. _____
3. _____ 6. _____

Weekly Summary (good/bad/other/weight/etc.)

Workout Summary & Diet Notes:

Sleep Hours

Daily Successes:

1.
2.
3.

TODAY'S GOALS

1.
2.
3.
4.

DONE?

○
○
○
○

Workout Summary & Diet Notes:

Sleep Hours

Daily Successes:

1.
2.
3.

TODAY'S GOALS

1.
2.
3.
4.

DONE?

○
○
○
○

Workout Summary & Diet Notes:

Sleep Hours

Daily Successes:

1.
2.
3.

TODAY'S GOALS

1.
2.
3.
4.

DONE?

○
○
○
○

Fitness Highlights of this Week

1.
2.
3.
4.
5.

Weekly Fitness Notes

RHR

BP

Total Distance (in miles)

Week

Year

Weight

WEEK 5

You Are Your Own Gym

I already said a good amount about this book in the Exercise section so I won't bore you with repeating most of it, but I include this toward the top of the Suggested Reading List because I believe the sooner you start using it, the happier you'll be and the quicker the results will begin. It's a highly effective tool in setting up workouts for yourself that are completely free of any external needs, and you can put it to use anywhere you are at any time. It's like having an on-demand personal trainer that isn't charging big bucks per hour and is ready to go anytime you are, 24/7!

I also like the fact that this has progressing difficulty stages which means that the book will work at your current level and still be just as useful as you get stronger, more resilient and are looking to increase the challenge and intensity. It's a lot of bang for your buck ($13 new and $6 used from Amazon) and a book you can use for years, as I know from experience. Also helpful is the included schedules, which provide the suggested workout for each day for whatever program you're doing that week.

WEEK 6

Date: _____

MONDAY
Day in review - What made today memorable?

TUESDAY
Day in review - What made today memorable?

WEDNESDAY
Day in review - What made today memorable?

THURSDAY
Day in review - What made today memorable?

"Think like a man of action; act like a man of thought." — *Henri Bergson*

Workout Summary & Diet Notes:	TODAY'S GOALS	DONE?
Sleep Hours	1.	◯
	2.	◯
Daily Successes:	3.	◯
1.	4.	◯
2.		
3.		

Workout Summary & Diet Notes:	TODAY'S GOALS	DONE?
Sleep Hours	1.	◯
	2.	◯
Daily Successes:	3.	◯
1.	4.	◯
2.		
3.		

Workout Summary & Diet Notes:	TODAY'S GOALS	DONE?
Sleep Hours	1.	◯
	2.	◯
Daily Successes:	3.	◯
1.	4.	◯
2.		
3.		

Workout Summary & Diet Notes:	TODAY'S GOALS	DONE?
Sleep Hours	1.	◯
	2.	◯
Daily Successes:	3.	◯
1.	4.	◯
2.		
3.		

FRIDAY

Day in review - What made today memorable?

SATURDAY

Day in review - What made today memorable?

SUNDAY

Day in review - What made today memorable?

Highlights of this Week

1.
2.
3.
4.
5.

Reminder From Your Past Self

Top Priorities For Next Week

1.   4.
2.   5.
3.   6.

Weekly Summary (good/bad/other/weight/etc.)

Workout Summary & Diet Notes:

Sleep
Hours

Daily Successes:

1.
2.
3.

TODAY'S GOALS

1.
2.
3.
4.

DONE?

○
○
○
○

Workout Summary & Diet Notes:

Sleep
Hours

Daily Successes:

1.
2.
3.

TODAY'S GOALS

1.
2.
3.
4.

DONE?

○
○
○
○

Workout Summary & Diet Notes:

Sleep
Hours

Daily Successes:

1.
2.
3.

TODAY'S GOALS

1.
2.
3.
4.

DONE?

○
○
○
○

Fitness Highlights of this Week

1.
2.
3.
4.
5.

Weekly Fitness Notes

RHR

BP

Total Distance
(in miles)

Week   Year

Weight

WEEK 6

WEEK 7

Date: _____

MONDAY

Day in review - What made today memorable?

TUESDAY

Day in review - What made today memorable?

WEDNESDAY

Day in review - What made today memorable?

THURSDAY

Day in review - What made today memorable?

"It is better to fail in originality than to succeed in imitation."
— *Herman Melville*

Workout Summary & Diet Notes:	TODAY'S GOALS	DONE?
Sleep Hours	1. _____	◯
	2. _____	◯
Daily Successes:	3. _____	◯
1. _____	4. _____	◯
2. _____		
3. _____		

Workout Summary & Diet Notes:	TODAY'S GOALS	DONE?
Sleep Hours	1. _____	◯
	2. _____	◯
Daily Successes:	3. _____	◯
1. _____	4. _____	◯
2. _____		
3. _____		

Workout Summary & Diet Notes:	TODAY'S GOALS	DONE?
Sleep Hours	1. _____	◯
	2. _____	◯
Daily Successes:	3. _____	◯
1. _____	4. _____	◯
2. _____		
3. _____		

Workout Summary & Diet Notes:	TODAY'S GOALS	DONE?
Sleep Hours	1. _____	◯
	2. _____	◯
Daily Successes:	3. _____	◯
1. _____	4. _____	◯
2. _____		
3. _____		

FRIDAY

Day in review - What made today memorable?

SATURDAY

Day in review - What made today memorable?

SUNDAY

Day in review - What made today memorable?

Highlights of this Week

1. _____
2. _____
3. _____
4. _____
5. _____

Reminder From Your Past Self

Top Priorities For Next Week

1. _____   4. _____
2. _____   5. _____
3. _____   6. _____

Weekly Summary (good/bad/other/weight/etc.)

Workout Summary & Diet Notes:

Sleep Hours

Daily Successes:

1. _____
2. _____
3. _____

TODAY'S GOALS

1. _____
2. _____
3. _____
4. _____

DONE?

○
○
○
○

Workout Summary & Diet Notes:

Sleep Hours

Daily Successes:

1. _____
2. _____
3. _____

TODAY'S GOALS

1. _____
2. _____
3. _____
4. _____

DONE?

○
○
○
○

Workout Summary & Diet Notes:

Sleep Hours

Daily Successes:

1. _____
2. _____
3. _____

TODAY'S GOALS

1. _____
2. _____
3. _____
4. _____

DONE?

○
○
○
○

Fitness Highlights of this Week

1. _____
2. _____
3. _____
4. _____
5. _____

Weekly Fitness Notes

RHR

BP

Total Distance (in miles)

Week [ ]   Year [ ]

Weight [ ]

WEEK 7

WEEK 8

Date: _____

MONDAY

Day in review - What made today memorable?

TUESDAY

Day in review - What made today memorable?

WEDNESDAY

Day in review - What made today memorable?

THURSDAY

Day in review - What made today memorable?

> "The road to success and the road to failure are almost exactly the same."
> — *Colin R. Davis*

Workout Summary & Diet Notes:	TODAY'S GOALS	DONE?
Sleep Hours	1. _____	◯
	2. _____	◯
Daily Successes:	3. _____	◯
1. _____	4. _____	◯
2. _____		
3. _____		

Workout Summary & Diet Notes:	TODAY'S GOALS	DONE?
Sleep Hours	1. _____	◯
	2. _____	◯
Daily Successes:	3. _____	◯
1. _____	4. _____	◯
2. _____		
3. _____		

Workout Summary & Diet Notes:	TODAY'S GOALS	DONE?
Sleep Hours	1. _____	◯
	2. _____	◯
Daily Successes:	3. _____	◯
1. _____	4. _____	◯
2. _____		
3. _____		

Workout Summary & Diet Notes:	TODAY'S GOALS	DONE?
Sleep Hours	1. _____	◯
	2. _____	◯
Daily Successes:	3. _____	◯
1. _____	4. _____	◯
2. _____		
3. _____		

FRIDAY

Day in review - What made today memorable?

SATURDAY

Day in review - What made today memorable?

SUNDAY

Day in review - What made today memorable?

Highlights of this Week

1. _____
2. _____
3. _____
4. _____
5. _____

Reminder From Your Past Self

Top Priorities For Next Week

1. _____   4. _____
2. _____   5. _____
3. _____   6. _____

Weekly Summary (good/bad/other/weight/etc.)

Workout Summary & Diet Notes:

Sleep Hours

Daily Successes:

1.
2.
3.

TODAY'S GOALS

1.
2.
3.
4.

DONE?

○
○
○
○

Workout Summary & Diet Notes:

Sleep Hours

Daily Successes:

1.
2.
3.

TODAY'S GOALS

1.
2.
3.
4.

DONE?

○
○
○
○

Workout Summary & Diet Notes:

Sleep Hours

Daily Successes:

1.
2.
3.

TODAY'S GOALS

1.
2.
3.
4.

DONE?

○
○
○
○

Fitness Highlights of this Week

1.
2.
3.
4.
5.

Weekly Fitness Notes

RHR

BP

Total Distance
(in miles)

Week ____   Year ____

Weight

WEEK 8

WEEK 9

Date: _____

MONDAY

Day in review - What made today memorable?

TUESDAY

Day in review - What made today memorable?

WEDNESDAY

Day in review - What made today memorable?

THURSDAY

Day in review - What made today memorable?

> "Success usually comes to those who are too busy to be looking for it."
> — *Henry David Thoreau*

Workout Summary & Diet Notes:	TODAY'S GOALS	DONE?
Sleep Hours	1.	◯
	2.	◯
Daily Successes:	3.	◯
1.	4.	◯
2.		
3.		

Workout Summary & Diet Notes:	TODAY'S GOALS	DONE?
Sleep Hours	1.	◯
	2.	◯
Daily Successes:	3.	◯
1.	4.	◯
2.		
3.		

Workout Summary & Diet Notes:	TODAY'S GOALS	DONE?
Sleep Hours	1.	◯
	2.	◯
Daily Successes:	3.	◯
1.	4.	◯
2.		
3.		

Workout Summary & Diet Notes:	TODAY'S GOALS	DONE?
Sleep Hours	1.	◯
	2.	◯
Daily Successes:	3.	◯
1.	4.	◯
2.		
3.		

FRIDAY

Day in review - What made today memorable?

SATURDAY

Day in review - What made today memorable?

SUNDAY

Day in review - What made today memorable?

Highlights of this Week

1.
2.
3.
4.
5.

Reminder From Your Past Self

Top Priorities For Next Week

1.   4.
2.   5.
3.   6.

Weekly Summary (good/bad/other/weight/etc.)

Workout Summary & Diet Notes:

Sleep Hours

Daily Successes:

1.
2.
3.

TODAY'S GOALS

DONE?

1. ○
2. ○
3. ○
4. ○

Workout Summary & Diet Notes:

Sleep Hours

Daily Successes:

1.
2.
3.

TODAY'S GOALS

DONE?

1. ○
2. ○
3. ○
4. ○

Workout Summary & Diet Notes:

Sleep Hours

Daily Successes:

1.
2.
3.

TODAY'S GOALS

DONE?

1. ○
2. ○
3. ○
4. ○

Fitness Highlights of this Week

1.
2.
3.
4.
5.

Weekly Fitness Notes

RHR

BP

Total Distance (in miles)

Week [ ] Year [ ]

Weight [ ]

WEEK 9

On Target Living

C hris Johnson somehow manages to take the whole wide universe of diet and nutrition and condense everything you need to know into roughly 300 pages. With all of the information this book contains it would be easy for it to turn into a medical journal that would be anything but enjoyable to read, but Chris does a masterful job of delivering the content in a highly readable way. This book is a roadmap on not only how to improve your diet in all areas without torturing yourself (as I wrote about earlier pertaining to the Food Target) but also how our diet is directly connected to our overall health, wellness, and longevity. Aside from diet and nutrition (those two categories alone make this book something you will get a huge benefit from), *On Target Living* also covers quite a bit on stress reduction, life/work balance and how healthy living practices and what we eat apply to achieving further successes in other areas of our lives that aren't always thought to be connected.

WEEK 10

Date: _____

MONDAY

Day in review - What made today memorable?

TUESDAY

Day in review - What made today memorable?

WEDNESDAY

Day in review - What made today memorable?

THURSDAY

Day in review - What made today memorable?

"Opportunities don't happen. You create them." — *Chris Grosser*

Workout Summary & Diet Notes:	TODAY'S GOALS	DONE?
Sleep Hours	1. _____	◯
	2. _____	◯
Daily Successes:	3. _____	◯
1. _____	4. _____	◯
2. _____		
3. _____		

Workout Summary & Diet Notes:	TODAY'S GOALS	DONE?
Sleep Hours	1. _____	◯
	2. _____	◯
Daily Successes:	3. _____	◯
1. _____	4. _____	◯
2. _____		
3. _____		

Workout Summary & Diet Notes:	TODAY'S GOALS	DONE?
Sleep Hours	1. _____	◯
	2. _____	◯
Daily Successes:	3. _____	◯
1. _____	4. _____	◯
2. _____		
3. _____		

Sleep Hours

FRIDAY

Day in review - What made today memorable?

SATURDAY

Day in review - What made today memorable?

SUNDAY

Day in review - What made today memorable?

Highlights of this Week

1.
2.
3.
4.
5.

Reminder From Your Past Self

Top Priorities For Next Week

1.   4.
2.   5.
3.   6.

Weekly Summary (good/bad/other/weight/etc.)

Workout Summary & Diet Notes:	TODAY'S GOALS	DONE?
Sleep Hours	1.	◯
	2.	◯
Daily Successes:	3.	◯
1.	4.	◯
2.		
3.		

Workout Summary & Diet Notes:	TODAY'S GOALS	DONE?
Sleep Hours	1.	◯
	2.	◯
Daily Successes:	3.	◯
1.	4.	◯
2.		
3.		

Workout Summary & Diet Notes:	TODAY'S GOALS	DONE?
Sleep Hours	1.	◯
	2.	◯
Daily Successes:	3.	◯
1.	4.	◯
2.		
3.		

Fitness Highlights of this Week

1.
2.
3.
4.
5.

Weekly Fitness Notes

RHR

BP

Total Distance (in miles)

Week ___ Year ___

Weight ___

WEEK 10

WEEK 11

Date: _____

MONDAY
Day in review - What made today memorable?

TUESDAY
Day in review - What made today memorable?

WEDNESDAY
Day in review - What made today memorable?

THURSDAY
Day in review - What made today memorable?

"Don't be afraid to give up the good to go for the great."
— *John D. Rockefeller*

Workout Summary & Diet Notes:	TODAY'S GOALS	DONE?
Sleep Hours **Daily Successes:** 1. 2. 3.	1. _____ 2. _____ 3. _____ 4. _____	○ ○ ○ ○
Workout Summary & Diet Notes:	TODAY'S GOALS	DONE?
Sleep Hours **Daily Successes:** 1. 2. 3.	1. _____ 2. _____ 3. _____ 4. _____	○ ○ ○ ○
Workout Summary & Diet Notes:	TODAY'S GOALS	DONE?
Sleep Hours **Daily Successes:** 1. 2. 3.	1. _____ 2. _____ 3. _____ 4. _____	○ ○ ○ ○
Workout Summary & Diet Notes:	TODAY'S GOALS	DONE?
Sleep Hours **Daily Successes:** 1. 2. 3.	1. _____ 2. _____ 3. _____ 4. _____	○ ○ ○ ○

FRIDAY

Day in review - What made today memorable?

SATURDAY

Day in review - What made today memorable?

SUNDAY

Day in review - What made today memorable?

Highlights of this Week

1.
2.
3.
4.
5.

Top Priorities For Next Week

1.   4.
2.   5.
3.   6.

Weekly Summary (good/bad/other/weight/etc.)

Reminder From Your Past Self

Workout Summary & Diet Notes:

Sleep Hours

Daily Successes:

1.
2.
3.

TODAY'S GOALS

DONE?

1.
2.
3.
4.

Workout Summary & Diet Notes:

Sleep Hours

Daily Successes:

1.
2.
3.

TODAY'S GOALS

DONE?

1.
2.
3.
4.

Workout Summary & Diet Notes:

Sleep Hours

Daily Successes:

1.
2.
3.

TODAY'S GOALS

DONE?

1.
2.
3.
4.

Fitness Highlights of this Week

1.
2.
3.
4.
5.

Weekly Fitness Notes

RHR

BP

Total Distance
(in miles)

Week   Year

Weight

WEEK 11

WEEK 12

Date: _____

MONDAY

Day in review - What made today memorable?

TUESDAY

Day in review - What made today memorable?

WEDNESDAY

Day in review - What made today memorable?

THURSDAY

Day in review - What made today memorable?

"I find that the harder I work, the more luck I seem to have."
— *Thomas Jefferson*

Workout Summary & Diet Notes:	TODAY'S GOALS	DONE?
Sleep Hours	1.	◯
	2.	◯
Daily Successes:	3.	◯
1.	4.	◯
2.		
3.		

Workout Summary & Diet Notes:	TODAY'S GOALS	DONE?
Sleep Hours	1.	◯
	2.	◯
Daily Successes:	3.	◯
1.	4.	◯
2.		
3.		

Workout Summary & Diet Notes:	TODAY'S GOALS	DONE?
Sleep Hours	1.	◯
	2.	◯
Daily Successes:	3.	◯
1.	4.	◯
2.		
3.		

Workout Summary & Diet Notes:	TODAY'S GOALS	DONE?
Sleep Hours	1.	◯
	2.	◯
Daily Successes:	3.	◯
1.	4.	◯
2.		
3.		

FRIDAY

Day in review - What made today memorable?

SATURDAY

Day in review - What made today memorable?

SUNDAY

Day in review - What made today memorable?

Highlights of this Week

1.
2.
3.
4.
5.

Reminder From Your Past Self

Top Priorities For Next Week

1.   4.
2.   5.
3.   6.

Weekly Summary (good/bad/other/weight/etc.)

Workout Summary & Diet Notes:

Sleep Hours

Daily Successes:

1.
2.
3.

TODAY'S GOALS

1.
2.
3.
4.

DONE?

○
○
○
○

Workout Summary & Diet Notes:

Sleep Hours

Daily Successes:

1.
2.
3.

TODAY'S GOALS

1.
2.
3.
4.

DONE?

○
○
○
○

Workout Summary & Diet Notes:

Sleep Hours

Daily Successes:

1.
2.
3.

TODAY'S GOALS

1.
2.
3.
4.

DONE?

○
○
○
○

Fitness Highlights of this Week

1.
2.
3.
4.
5.

Weekly Fitness Notes

RHR

BP

Total Distance
(in miles)

Week ____   Year ____

Weight

WEEK 12

WEEK 13

Date: _____

MONDAY

Day in review - What made today memorable?

TUESDAY

Day in review - What made today memorable?

WEDNESDAY

Day in review - What made today memorable?

THURSDAY

Day in review - What made today memorable?

> "There are two types of people who will tell you that you cannot make a difference in this world: those who are afraid to try and those who are afraid you will succeed." — *Ray Goforth*

Workout Summary & Diet Notes:	TODAY'S GOALS	DONE?
Sleep Hours	1. _____	◯
	2. _____	◯
Daily Successes:	3. _____	◯
1. _____	4. _____	◯
2. _____		
3. _____		

Workout Summary & Diet Notes:	TODAY'S GOALS	DONE?
Sleep Hours	1. _____	◯
	2. _____	◯
Daily Successes:	3. _____	◯
1. _____	4. _____	◯
2. _____		
3. _____		

Workout Summary & Diet Notes:	TODAY'S GOALS	DONE?
Sleep Hours	1. _____	◯
	2. _____	◯
Daily Successes:	3. _____	◯
1. _____	4. _____	◯
2. _____		
3. _____		

Workout Summary & Diet Notes:	TODAY'S GOALS	DONE?
Sleep Hours	1. _____	◯
	2. _____	◯
Daily Successes:	3. _____	◯
1. _____	4. _____	◯
2. _____		
3. _____		

FRIDAY

Day in review – What made today memorable?

SATURDAY

Day in review – What made today memorable?

SUNDAY

Day in review – What made today memorable?

Highlights of this Week

1.
2.
3.
4.
5.

Top Priorities For Next Week

1.   4.
2.   5.
3.   6.

Weekly Summary (good/bad/other/weight/etc.)

Reminder From Your Past Self

Workout Summary & Diet Notes:

Sleep Hours

Daily Successes:
1.
2.
3.

TODAY'S GOALS | DONE?
1. ⭕
2. ⭕
3. ⭕
4. ⭕

Workout Summary & Diet Notes:

Sleep Hours

Daily Successes:
1.
2.
3.

TODAY'S GOALS | DONE?
1. ⭕
2. ⭕
3. ⭕
4. ⭕

Workout Summary & Diet Notes:

Sleep Hours

Daily Successes:
1.
2.
3.

TODAY'S GOALS | DONE?
1. ⭕
2. ⭕
3. ⭕
4. ⭕

Fitness Highlights of this Week
1.
2.
3.
4.
5.

Weekly Fitness Notes

RHR

BP

Total Distance (in miles)

Week | Year

Weight

WEEK 13

Emotional Intelligence 2.0

Emotional intelligence (aka EQ) as a central role in our overall success in life is a topic that has become increasingly researched and documented in the 11 years since this book came out, and not surprisingly all the additional interest has brought forth many more books on the subject. *Emotional Intelligence 2.0* was one of the originals and is still widely considered one of the best on the field. There is a lot of useful info in this book although some of the negative reviews are around the fact that it isn't longer and is too basic, but as a general starting point on the topic of EQ, I think the authors do a great job.

One point of note on how and where you get this book. Each book comes with a unique access code for an online EQ assessment. The concept is, you do the test at the beginning before you read the book and then once again at the end. Weak areas originally identified during your first assessment become specific areas of focus and improvement while you read the book. So if you buy this used or get it from the library that's fine, but you most likely won't be able to do the online assessment component as the code will be void.

WEEK 14

Date: _____

MONDAY
Day in review - What made today memorable?

TUESDAY
Day in review - What made today memorable?

WEDNESDAY
Day in review - What made today memorable?

THURSDAY
Day in review - What made today memorable?

"Twenty years from now you will be more disappointed by the things that you didn't do than by the ones you did do. So throw off the bowlines. Sail away from the safe harbor. Catch the trade winds in your sails. Explore. Dream. Discover." — *Mark Twain*

Workout Summary & Diet Notes:	TODAY'S GOALS	DONE?
Sleep Hours	1.	◯
	2.	◯
Daily Successes:	3.	◯
1.		
2.	4.	◯
3.		

Workout Summary & Diet Notes:	TODAY'S GOALS	DONE?
Sleep Hours	1.	◯
	2.	◯
Daily Successes:	3.	◯
1.		
2.	4.	◯
3.		

Workout Summary & Diet Notes:	TODAY'S GOALS	DONE?
Sleep Hours	1.	◯
	2.	◯
Daily Successes:	3.	◯
1.		
2.	4.	◯
3.		

Workout Summary & Diet Notes:	TODAY'S GOALS	DONE?
Sleep Hours	1.	◯
	2.	◯
Daily Successes:	3.	◯
1.		
2.	4.	◯
3.		

FRIDAY

Day in review - What made today memorable?

SATURDAY

Day in review - What made today memorable?

SUNDAY

Day in review - What made today memorable?

Highlights of this Week

1. _____
2. _____
3. _____
4. _____
5. _____

Reminder From Your Past Self

Top Priorities For Next Week

1. _____ 4. _____
2. _____ 5. _____
3. _____ 6. _____

Weekly Summary (good/bad/other/weight/etc.)

Workout Summary & Diet Notes:

Sleep
Hours

Daily Successes:

1. _____
2. _____
3. _____

TODAY'S GOALS

1. _____
2. _____
3. _____
4. _____

DONE?

○
○
○
○

Workout Summary & Diet Notes:

Sleep
Hours

Daily Successes:

1. _____
2. _____
3. _____

TODAY'S GOALS

1. _____
2. _____
3. _____
4. _____

DONE?

○
○
○
○

Workout Summary & Diet Notes:

Sleep
Hours

Daily Successes:

1. _____
2. _____
3. _____

TODAY'S GOALS

1. _____
2. _____
3. _____
4. _____

DONE?

○
○
○
○

Fitness Highlights of this Week

1. _____
2. _____
3. _____
4. _____
5. _____

Weekly Fitness Notes

RHR

BP

Total Distance (in miles)

Week [ ] Year [ ]

Weight [ ]

WEEK 14

WEEK 15

Date: _____

MONDAY

Day in review - What made today memorable?

TUESDAY

Day in review - What made today memorable?

WEDNESDAY

Day in review - What made today memorable?

THURSDAY

Day in review - What made today memorable?

"Be not afraid of growing slowly; be afraid only of standing still."
— Chinese Proverb

Workout Summary & Diet Notes:	TODAY'S GOALS	DONE?
Sleep Hours **Daily Successes:** 1. _____ 2. _____ 3. _____	1. _____ 2. _____ 3. _____ 4. _____	○ ○ ○ ○

Workout Summary & Diet Notes:	TODAY'S GOALS	DONE?
Sleep Hours **Daily Successes:** 1. _____ 2. _____ 3. _____	1. _____ 2. _____ 3. _____ 4. _____	○ ○ ○ ○

Workout Summary & Diet Notes:	TODAY'S GOALS	DONE?
Sleep Hours **Daily Successes:** 1. _____ 2. _____ 3. _____	1. _____ 2. _____ 3. _____ 4. _____	○ ○ ○ ○

Workout Summary & Diet Notes:	TODAY'S GOALS	DONE?
Sleep Hours **Daily Successes:** 1. _____ 2. _____ 3. _____	1. _____ 2. _____ 3. _____ 4. _____	○ ○ ○ ○

FRIDAY

Day in review - What made today memorable?

SATURDAY

Day in review - What made today memorable?

SUNDAY

Day in review - What made today memorable?

Highlights of this Week

1.
2.
3.
4.
5.

Reminder From Your Past Self

Top Priorities For Next Week

1.   4.
2.   5.
3.   6.

Weekly Summary (good/bad/other/weight/etc.)

Workout Summary & Diet Notes:

Sleep Hours

Daily Successes:

1.
2.
3.

TODAY'S GOALS

DONE?

1.
2.
3.
4.

Workout Summary & Diet Notes:

Sleep Hours

Daily Successes:

1.
2.
3.

TODAY'S GOALS

DONE?

1.
2.
3.
4.

Workout Summary & Diet Notes:

Sleep Hours

Daily Successes:

1.
2.
3.

TODAY'S GOALS

DONE?

1.
2.
3.
4.

Fitness Highlights of this Week

1.
2.
3.
4.
5.

Weekly Fitness Notes

RHR

BP

Total Distance (in miles)

Week

Year

Weight

WEEK 15

WEEK 16

Date: _____

MONDAY

Day in review - What made today memorable?

TUESDAY

Day in review - What made today memorable?

WEDNESDAY

Day in review - What made today memorable?

THURSDAY

Day in review - What made today memorable?

> "The will to win, the desire to succeed, the urge to reach your full potential
> . . . these are the keys that will unlock the door to personal excellence."
> — *Confucius*

Workout Summary & Diet Notes:	TODAY'S GOALS	DONE?
Sleep Hours	1.	◯
	2.	◯
Daily Successes:	3.	◯
1.	4.	◯
2.		
3.		

Workout Summary & Diet Notes:	TODAY'S GOALS	DONE?
Sleep Hours	1.	◯
	2.	◯
Daily Successes:	3.	◯
1.	4.	◯
2.		
3.		

Workout Summary & Diet Notes:	TODAY'S GOALS	DONE?
Sleep Hours	1.	◯
	2.	◯
Daily Successes:	3.	◯
1.	4.	◯
2.		
3.		

Workout Summary & Diet Notes:	TODAY'S GOALS	DONE?
Sleep Hours	1.	◯
	2.	◯
Daily Successes:	3.	◯
1.	4.	◯
2.		
3.		

FRIDAY

Day in review - What made today memorable?

SATURDAY

Day in review - What made today memorable?

SUNDAY

Day in review - What made today memorable?

Highlights of this Week

1. _____
2. _____
3. _____
4. _____
5. _____

Top Priorities For Next Week

1. _____   4. _____
2. _____   5. _____
3. _____   6. _____

Reminder From Your Past Self

Weekly Summary (good/bad/other/weight/etc.)

Workout Summary & Diet Notes:

Sleep Hours

Daily Successes:

1.
2.
3.

TODAY'S GOALS

1.
2.
3.
4.

DONE?

○
○
○
○

Workout Summary & Diet Notes:

Sleep Hours

Daily Successes:

1.
2.
3.

TODAY'S GOALS

1.
2.
3.
4.

DONE?

○
○
○
○

Workout Summary & Diet Notes:

Sleep Hours

Daily Successes:

1.
2.
3.

TODAY'S GOALS

1.
2.
3.
4.

DONE?

○
○
○
○

Fitness Highlights of this Week

1.
2.
3.
4.
5.

Weekly Fitness Notes

RHR

BP

Total Distance (in miles)

Week

Year

Weight

WEEK 16

WEEK 17

Date: _____

MONDAY

Day in review - What made today memorable?

TUESDAY

Day in review - What made today memorable?

WEDNESDAY

Day in review - What made today memorable?

THURSDAY

Day in review - What made today memorable?

"We are products of our past, but we don't have to be prisoners of it."
— *Rick Warren*

Workout Summary & Diet Notes:	TODAY'S GOALS	DONE?
Sleep Hours	1. _____	◯
	2. _____	◯
Daily Successes:	3. _____	◯
1. _____	4. _____	◯
2. _____		
3. _____		

Workout Summary & Diet Notes:	TODAY'S GOALS	DONE?
Sleep Hours	1. _____	◯
	2. _____	◯
Daily Successes:	3. _____	◯
1. _____	4. _____	◯
2. _____		
3. _____		

Workout Summary & Diet Notes:	TODAY'S GOALS	DONE?
Sleep Hours	1. _____	◯
	2. _____	◯
Daily Successes:	3. _____	◯
1. _____	4. _____	◯
2. _____		
3. _____		

Workout Summary & Diet Notes:	TODAY'S GOALS	DONE?
Sleep Hours	1. _____	◯
	2. _____	◯
Daily Successes:	3. _____	◯
1. _____	4. _____	◯
2. _____		
3. _____		

FRIDAY

Day in review - What made today memorable?

SATURDAY

Day in review - What made today memorable?

SUNDAY

Day in review - What made today memorable?

Highlights of this Week

1.
2.
3.
4.
5.

Reminder From Your Past Self

Top Priorities For Next Week

1.
2.
3.
4.
5.
6.

Weekly Summary (good/bad/other/weight/etc.)

Workout Summary & Diet Notes:

Sleep Hours

Daily Successes:

1.
2.
3.

TODAY'S GOALS

DONE?

1.
2.
3.
4.

○ ○ ○ ○

Workout Summary & Diet Notes:

Sleep Hours

Daily Successes:

1.
2.
3.

TODAY'S GOALS

DONE?

1.
2.
3.
4.

○ ○ ○ ○

Workout Summary & Diet Notes:

Sleep Hours

Daily Successes:

1.
2.
3.

TODAY'S GOALS

DONE?

1.
2.
3.
4.

○ ○ ○ ○

Fitness Highlights of this Week

1.
2.
3.
4.
5.

Weekly Fitness Notes

RHR

BP

Total Distance (in miles)

Week [ ] Year [ ]

Weight [ ]

WEEK 17

Incognito

One of the reasons this book stands out is the amount of neuroscience knowledge it will give you in the form of an entertaining summer beach book. Reading this you will gain a ton of useful info about the inner workings of the brain and exploration of everything that is happening within. If the conscious part of our thinking is just the "tip of the iceberg" of what our mind is doing, then this book provides something of a guided tour of everything below the surface. "David Eagleman reveals all the neural magic tricks behind the cognitive illusion of reality" as Jonah Lehrer (author of *How We Decide*) puts it.

Eagleman is a neuroscientist at Baylor College of Medicine so he certainly has the expert credentials to deliver the facts and insights that make this book so informative, but he also is a fiction author which is evident in his ability to hold a reader's attention hostage for long stretches at a time. I had this book on a flight from Philly to California and the six-hour trip went by in a blink.

WEEK 18

Date: _____

MONDAY

Day in review - What made today memorable?

TUESDAY

Day in review - What made today memorable?

WEDNESDAY

Day in review - What made today memorable?

THURSDAY

Day in review - What made today memorable?

"If you don't make the time to work on creating the life you want, you're eventually going to be forced to spend a lot of time dealing with a life you don't want." — *Kevin Ngo*

Workout Summary & Diet Notes:	TODAY'S GOALS	DONE?
Sleep Hours	1.	○
	2.	○
Daily Successes:	3.	○
1.	4.	○
2.		
3.		

Workout Summary & Diet Notes:	TODAY'S GOALS	DONE?
Sleep Hours	1.	○
	2.	○
Daily Successes:	3.	○
1.	4.	○
2.		
3.		

Workout Summary & Diet Notes:	TODAY'S GOALS	DONE?
Sleep Hours	1.	○
	2.	○
Daily Successes:	3.	○
1.	4.	○
2.		
3.		

Workout Summary & Diet Notes:	TODAY'S GOALS	DONE?
Sleep Hours	1.	○
	2.	○
Daily Successes:	3.	○
1.	4.	○
2.		
3.		

FRIDAY

Day in review - What made today memorable?

SATURDAY

Day in review - What made today memorable?

SUNDAY

Day in review - What made today memorable?

Highlights of this Week

1.
2.
3.
4.
5.

Top Priorities For Next Week

1.   4.
2.   5.
3.   6.

Weekly Summary (good/bad/other/weight/etc.)

Reminder From Your Past Self

Workout Summary & Diet Notes:

Sleep
Hours

Daily Successes:

1.
2.
3.

TODAY'S GOALS

1.
2.
3.
4.

DONE?

○
○
○
○

Workout Summary & Diet Notes:

Sleep
Hours

Daily Successes:

1.
2.
3.

TODAY'S GOALS

1.
2.
3.
4.

DONE?

○
○
○
○

Workout Summary & Diet Notes:

Sleep
Hours

Daily Successes:

1.
2.
3.

TODAY'S GOALS

1.
2.
3.
4.

DONE?

○
○
○
○

Fitness Highlights of this Week

1.
2.
3.
4.
5.

Weekly Fitness Notes

RHR

BP

Total Distance
(in miles)

Week   Year

Weight

WEEK 18

WEEK 19

Date: _____

MONDAY

Day in review - What made today memorable?

TUESDAY

Day in review - What made today memorable?

WEDNESDAY

Day in review - What made today memorable?

THURSDAY

Day in review - What made today memorable?

"The tragedy in life doesn't lie in not reaching your goal. The tragedy lies in having no goal to reach." — *Benjamin Mays*

Workout Summary & Diet Notes:	TODAY'S GOALS	DONE?
Sleep Hours	1.	○
	2.	○
Daily Successes:	3.	○
1.	4.	○
2.		
3.		

Workout Summary & Diet Notes:	TODAY'S GOALS	DONE?
Sleep Hours	1.	○
	2.	○
Daily Successes:	3.	○
1.	4.	○
2.		
3.		

Workout Summary & Diet Notes:	TODAY'S GOALS	DONE?
Sleep Hours	1.	○
	2.	○
Daily Successes:	3.	○
1.	4.	○
2.		
3.		

Workout Summary & Diet Notes:	TODAY'S GOALS	DONE?
Sleep Hours	1.	○
	2.	○
Daily Successes:	3.	○
1.	4.	○
2.		
3.		

FRIDAY

Day in review - What made today memorable?

SATURDAY

Day in review - What made today memorable?

SUNDAY

Day in review - What made today memorable?

Highlights of this Week

1.
2.
3.
4.
5.

Top Priorities For Next Week

1.   4.
2.   5.
3.   6.

Reminder From Your Past Self

Weekly Summary (good/bad/other/weight/etc.)

Workout Summary & Diet Notes:

Sleep Hours

Daily Successes:

1.
2.
3.

TODAY'S GOALS

1.
2.
3.
4.

DONE?

○
○
○
○

Workout Summary & Diet Notes:

Sleep Hours

Daily Successes:

1.
2.
3.

TODAY'S GOALS

1.
2.
3.
4.

DONE?

○
○
○
○

Workout Summary & Diet Notes:

Sleep Hours

Daily Successes:

1.
2.
3.

TODAY'S GOALS

1.
2.
3.
4.

DONE?

○
○
○
○

Fitness Highlights of this Week

1.
2.
3.
4.
5.

Weekly Fitness Notes

RHR

BP

Total Distance (in miles)

Week

Year

Weight

WEEK 19

WEEK 20

Date: _____

MONDAY

Day in review - What made today memorable?

TUESDAY

Day in review - What made today memorable?

WEDNESDAY

Day in review - What made today memorable?

THURSDAY

Day in review - What made today memorable?

"With self-discipline most anything is possible." — *Theodore Roosevelt*

Workout Summary & Diet Notes:	TODAY'S GOALS	DONE?
Sleep Hours	1.	◯
	2.	◯
Daily Successes:	3.	◯
1.	4.	◯
2.		
3.		

Workout Summary & Diet Notes:	TODAY'S GOALS	DONE?
Sleep Hours	1.	◯
	2.	◯
Daily Successes:	3.	◯
1.	4.	◯
2.		
3.		

Workout Summary & Diet Notes:	TODAY'S GOALS	DONE?
Sleep Hours	1.	◯
	2.	◯
Daily Successes:	3.	◯
1.	4.	◯
2.		
3.		

Workout Summary & Diet Notes:	TODAY'S GOALS	DONE?
Sleep Hours	1.	◯
	2.	◯
Daily Successes:	3.	◯
1.	4.	◯
2.		
3.		

FRIDAY

Day in review - What made today memorable?

SATURDAY

Day in review - What made today memorable?

SUNDAY

Day in review - What made today memorable?

Highlights of this Week

1. _____
2. _____
3. _____
4. _____
5. _____

Top Priorities For Next Week

1. _____ 4. _____
2. _____ 5. _____
3. _____ 6. _____

Weekly Summary (good/bad/other/weight/etc.)

Reminder From Your Past Self

Workout Summary & Diet Notes:

Sleep Hours

Daily Successes:
1.
2.
3.

TODAY'S GOALS

1.
2.
3.
4.

DONE?

○
○
○
○

Workout Summary & Diet Notes:

Sleep Hours

Daily Successes:
1.
2.
3.

TODAY'S GOALS

1.
2.
3.
4.

DONE?

○
○
○
○

Workout Summary & Diet Notes:

Sleep Hours

Daily Successes:
1.
2.
3.

TODAY'S GOALS

1.
2.
3.
4.

DONE?

○
○
○
○

Fitness Highlights of this Week

1.
2.
3.
4.
5.

Weekly Fitness Notes

RHR

BP

Total Distance (in miles)

Week ___ Year ___

Weight

WEEK 20

WEEK 21

Date: _____

MONDAY

Day in review - What made today memorable?

TUESDAY

Day in review - What made today memorable?

WEDNESDAY

Day in review - What made today memorable?

THURSDAY

Day in review - What made today memorable?

> "Success is simple. Do what's right, the right way, at the right time."
> — *Arnold H. Glasgow*

Workout Summary & Diet Notes:	TODAY'S GOALS	DONE?
Sleep Hours **Daily Successes:** 1. ____ 2. ____ 3. ____	1. ____ 2. ____ 3. ____ 4. ____	○ ○ ○ ○
Sleep Hours **Daily Successes:** 1. ____ 2. ____ 3. ____	1. ____ 2. ____ 3. ____ 4. ____	○ ○ ○ ○
Sleep Hours **Daily Successes:** 1. ____ 2. ____ 3. ____	1. ____ 2. ____ 3. ____ 4. ____	○ ○ ○ ○
Sleep Hours **Daily Successes:** 1. ____ 2. ____ 3. ____	1. ____ 2. ____ 3. ____ 4. ____	○ ○ ○ ○

FRIDAY

Day in review - What made today memorable?

SATURDAY

Day in review - What made today memorable?

SUNDAY

Day in review - What made today memorable?

Highlights of this Week

1.
2.
3.
4.
5.

Top Priorities For Next Week

1.   4.
2.   5.
3.   6.

Weekly Summary (good/bad/other/weight/etc.)

Reminder From Your Past Self

Workout Summary & Diet Notes:

Sleep Hours

Daily Successes:

1.
2.
3.

TODAY'S GOALS

1.
2.
3.
4.

DONE?

○
○
○
○

Workout Summary & Diet Notes:

Sleep Hours

Daily Successes:

1.
2.
3.

TODAY'S GOALS

1.
2.
3.
4.

DONE?

○
○
○
○

Workout Summary & Diet Notes:

Sleep Hours

Daily Successes:

1.
2.
3.

TODAY'S GOALS

1.
2.
3.
4.

DONE?

○
○
○
○

Fitness Highlights of this Week

1.
2.
3.
4.
5.

Weekly Fitness Notes

RHR

BP

Total Distance (in miles)

Week

Year

Weight

WEEK 21

Why We Sleep

I'm so convinced that you will have enjoyed *Incognito* that I added another neuroscientist author's immensely entertaining and educational book for this next month: *Why We Sleep*. A literary double header of brain science! This time it's Matthew Walker's excellent research findings on the largely uncharted wilderness that we spend roughly a third of our lives in: sleep.

Walker is a professor of Neuroscience at Berkeley, the Director of the Center for Human Sleep Science, a former professor of psychiatry at Harvard University . . . and a man passionate about the immense power and importance of sleep. This book not only explores and explains how we can harness that power to make the most of our waking hours, but provides all sorts of insights, examples and tools on how we can use sleep to become more successful in our careers, make better decisions, optimize physical performance, and regulate moods. Another aspect of this book I think you'll agree is pretty fascinating stuff is the cutting-edge research done around the study of dreams and how this "overnight therapy" works.

WEEK 22

Date: _____

MONDAY

Day in review - What made today memorable?

TUESDAY

Day in review - What made today memorable?

WEDNESDAY

Day in review - What made today memorable?

THURSDAY

Day in review - What made today memorable?

"Action is the foundational key to all success." — *Pablo Picasso*

Workout Summary & Diet Notes:	TODAY'S GOALS	DONE?
Sleep Hours	1.	○
	2.	○
Daily Successes:	3.	○
1.	4.	○
2.		
3.		

Workout Summary & Diet Notes:	TODAY'S GOALS	DONE?
Sleep Hours	1.	○
	2.	○
Daily Successes:	3.	○
1.	4.	○
2.		
3.		

Workout Summary & Diet Notes:	TODAY'S GOALS	DONE?
Sleep Hours	1.	○
	2.	○
Daily Successes:	3.	○
1.	4.	○
2.		
3.		

Workout Summary & Diet Notes:	TODAY'S GOALS	DONE?
Sleep Hours	1.	○
	2.	○
Daily Successes:	3.	○
1.	4.	○
2.		
3.		

FRIDAY

Day in review - What made today memorable?

SATURDAY

Day in review - What made today memorable?

SUNDAY

Day in review - What made today memorable?

Highlights of this Week

1.
2.
3.
4.
5.

Reminder From Your Past Self

Top Priorities For Next Week

1.   4.
2.   5.
3.   6.

Weekly Summary (good/bad/other/weight/etc.)

Workout Summary & Diet Notes:

Sleep Hours

Daily Successes:

1.
2.
3.

TODAY'S GOALS

1.
2.
3.
4.

DONE?

○
○
○
○

Workout Summary & Diet Notes:

Sleep Hours

Daily Successes:

1.
2.
3.

TODAY'S GOALS

1.
2.
3.
4.

DONE?

○
○
○
○

Workout Summary & Diet Notes:

Sleep Hours

Daily Successes:

1.
2.
3.

TODAY'S GOALS

1.
2.
3.
4.

DONE?

○
○
○
○

Fitness Highlights of this Week

1.
2.
3.
4.
5.

Weekly Fitness Notes

RHR

BP

Total Distance (in miles)

Week

Year

Weight

WEEK 22

WEEK 23

Date: _____

MONDAY

Day in review - What made today memorable?

TUESDAY

Day in review - What made today memorable?

WEDNESDAY

Day in review - What made today memorable?

THURSDAY

Day in review - What made today memorable?

> "The best years of your life are the ones in which you decide your problems are your own. You do not blame them on your mother, the ecology, or the president. You realize that you control your own destiny." — *Albert Ellis*

Workout Summary & Diet Notes:	**TODAY'S GOALS**	**DONE?**
Sleep Hours	1. _____	◯
	2. _____	◯
Daily Successes:	3. _____	◯
1. _____	4. _____	◯
2. _____		
3. _____		

Workout Summary & Diet Notes:	**TODAY'S GOALS**	**DONE?**
Sleep Hours	1. _____	◯
	2. _____	◯
Daily Successes:	3. _____	◯
1. _____	4. _____	◯
2. _____		
3. _____		

Workout Summary & Diet Notes:	**TODAY'S GOALS**	**DONE?**
Sleep Hours	1. _____	◯
	2. _____	◯
Daily Successes:	3. _____	◯
1. _____	4. _____	◯
2. _____		
3. _____		

Workout Summary & Diet Notes:	**TODAY'S GOALS**	**DONE?**
Sleep Hours	1. _____	◯
	2. _____	◯
Daily Successes:	3. _____	◯
1. _____	4. _____	◯
2. _____		
3. _____		

FRIDAY

Day in review - What made today memorable?

SATURDAY

Day in review - What made today memorable?

SUNDAY

Day in review - What made today memorable?

Highlights of this Week

1. _____
2. _____
3. _____
4. _____
5. _____

Reminder From Your Past Self

Top Priorities For Next Week

1. _____   4. _____
2. _____   5. _____
3. _____   6. _____

Weekly Summary (good/bad/other/weight/etc.)

Workout Summary & Diet Notes:

Sleep Hours

Daily Successes:

1. _____
2. _____
3. _____

TODAY'S GOALS

1. _____
2. _____
3. _____
4. _____

DONE?

◯
◯
◯
◯

Workout Summary & Diet Notes:

Sleep Hours

Daily Successes:

1. _____
2. _____
3. _____

TODAY'S GOALS

1. _____
2. _____
3. _____
4. _____

DONE?

◯
◯
◯
◯

Workout Summary & Diet Notes:

Sleep Hours

Daily Successes:

1. _____
2. _____
3. _____

TODAY'S GOALS

1. _____
2. _____
3. _____
4. _____

DONE?

◯
◯
◯
◯

Fitness Highlights of this Week

1. _____
2. _____
3. _____
4. _____
5. _____

Weekly Fitness Notes

RHR

BP

Total Distance (in miles)

Week [ ] Year [ ]

Weight [ ]

WEEK 23

WEEK 24

Date: _____

MONDAY
Day in review - What made today memorable?

TUESDAY
Day in review - What made today memorable?

WEDNESDAY
Day in review - What made today memorable?

THURSDAY
Day in review - What made today memorable?

"Success is going from failure to failure without losing enthusiasm."
— *Winston Churchill*

Workout Summary & Diet Notes:	TODAY'S GOALS	DONE?
Sleep Hours **Daily Successes:** 1. 2. 3.	1. 2. 3. 4.	◯ ◯ ◯ ◯

Workout Summary & Diet Notes:	TODAY'S GOALS	DONE?
Sleep Hours **Daily Successes:** 1. 2. 3.	1. 2. 3. 4.	◯ ◯ ◯ ◯

Workout Summary & Diet Notes:	TODAY'S GOALS	DONE?
Sleep Hours **Daily Successes:** 1. 2. 3.	1. 2. 3. 4.	◯ ◯ ◯ ◯

Workout Summary & Diet Notes:	TODAY'S GOALS	DONE?
Sleep Hours **Daily Successes:** 1. 2. 3.	1. 2. 3. 4.	◯ ◯ ◯ ◯

FRIDAY

Day in review - What made today memorable?

SATURDAY

Day in review - What made today memorable?

SUNDAY

Day in review - What made today memorable?

Highlights of this Week

1.
2.
3.
4.
5.

Reminder From Your Past Self

Top Priorities For Next Week

1.   4.
2.   5.
3.   6.

Weekly Summary (good/bad/other/weight/etc.)

Workout Summary & Diet Notes:

Sleep Hours

Daily Successes:

1.
2.
3.

TODAY'S GOALS

1.
2.
3.
4.

DONE?

○
○
○
○

Workout Summary & Diet Notes:

Sleep Hours

Daily Successes:

1.
2.
3.

TODAY'S GOALS

1.
2.
3.
4.

DONE?

○
○
○
○

Workout Summary & Diet Notes:

Daily Successes:

1.
2.
3.

TODAY'S GOALS

1.
2.
3.
4.

DONE?

○
○
○
○

Fitness Highlights of this Week

1.
2.
3.
4.
5.

Weekly Fitness Notes

RHR

BP

Total Distance (in miles)

Week

Year

Weight

WEEK 24

WEEK 25

Date: _____

MONDAY

Day in review - What made today memorable?

TUESDAY

Day in review - What made today memorable?

WEDNESDAY

Day in review - What made today memorable?

THURSDAY

Day in review - What made today memorable?

"If you want to make an easy job seem mighty hard, just keep putting off doing it." — *Olin Miller*

Workout Summary & Diet Notes:	TODAY'S GOALS	DONE?
Sleep Hours **Daily Successes:** 1. 2. 3.	1. _____ 2. _____ 3. _____ 4. _____	○ ○ ○ ○
Workout Summary & Diet Notes:	**TODAY'S GOALS**	**DONE?**
Sleep Hours **Daily Successes:** 1. 2. 3.	1. _____ 2. _____ 3. _____ 4. _____	○ ○ ○ ○
Workout Summary & Diet Notes:	**TODAY'S GOALS**	**DONE?**
Sleep Hours **Daily Successes:** 1. 2. 3.	1. _____ 2. _____ 3. _____ 4. _____	○ ○ ○ ○
Workout Summary & Diet Notes:	**TODAY'S GOALS**	**DONE?**
Sleep Hours **Daily Successes:** 1. 2. 3.	1. _____ 2. _____ 3. _____ 4. _____	○ ○ ○ ○

FRIDAY

Day in review - What made today memorable?

SATURDAY

Day in review - What made today memorable?

SUNDAY

Day in review - What made today memorable?

Highlights of this Week

1. _____
2. _____
3. _____
4. _____
5. _____

Reminder From Your Past Self

Top Priorities For Next Week

1. _____ 4. _____
2. _____ 5. _____
3. _____ 6. _____

Weekly Summary (good/bad/other/weight/etc.)

Workout Summary & Diet Notes:

Sleep Hours

Daily Successes:
1.
2.
3.

TODAY'S GOALS

1.
2.
3.
4.

DONE?

○
○
○
○

Workout Summary & Diet Notes:

Sleep Hours

Daily Successes:
1.
2.
3.

TODAY'S GOALS

1.
2.
3.
4.

DONE?

○
○
○
○

Workout Summary & Diet Notes:

Sleep Hours

Daily Successes:
1.
2.
3.

TODAY'S GOALS

1.
2.
3.
4.

DONE?

○
○
○
○

Fitness Highlights of this Week

1.
2.
3.
4.
5.

Weekly Fitness Notes

RHR

BP

Total Distance (in miles)

Week

Year

Weight

WEEK 25

Getting Things Done

Now that you are roughly at the halfway point of BAR40 my prediction is that you have been finding plenty of ways to improve your life in all areas and are continuously coming up with new ideas and goals that you want to implement. While this boost in productivity and motivation are fantastic developments, the resulting challenge can be how to best manage the increasingly crowded to-do list.

David Allen has the answers and system for you. You may have heard of him or his "GTD" (Getting Things Done) approach before as he is a bit of a time-management rock star and has gained a lot of attention in the business world for streamlining processes and increasing productivity. Think of this GTD book as a master's class in Project Management for your personal life, as well as however you may want to apply it in your career.

GTD ultimately is helping declutter, prioritize, sort, and manage every new task that gets tossed our way every day. Not only does the approach and system help avoid those overwhelmed thoughts of, where do I even start with this list! but also maximizes the quality of the output on each thing we are working on. Even a few techniques from this book that stay with you will make a big impact on your life.

WEEK 26

Date: _____

MONDAY

Day in review - What made today memorable?

TUESDAY

Day in review - What made today memorable?

WEDNESDAY

Day in review - What made today memorable?

THURSDAY

Day in review - What made today memorable?

"I attribute my success to this: I never gave or took any excuse."
— Florence Nightingale

Workout Summary & Diet Notes:	TODAY'S GOALS	DONE?
Sleep Hours	1. _____	○
	2. _____	○
Daily Successes:	3. _____	○
1. _____		
2. _____	4. _____	○
3. _____		

Workout Summary & Diet Notes:	TODAY'S GOALS	DONE?
Sleep Hours	1. _____	○
	2. _____	○
Daily Successes:	3. _____	○
1. _____		
2. _____	4. _____	○
3. _____		

Workout Summary & Diet Notes:	TODAY'S GOALS	DONE?
Sleep Hours	1. _____	○
	2. _____	○
Daily Successes:	3. _____	○
1. _____		
2. _____	4. _____	○
3. _____		

Workout Summary & Diet Notes:	TODAY'S GOALS	DONE?
Sleep Hours	1. _____	○
	2. _____	○
Daily Successes:	3. _____	○
1. _____		
2. _____	4. _____	○
3. _____		

FRIDAY

Day in review - What made today memorable?

SATURDAY

Day in review - What made today memorable?

SUNDAY

Day in review - What made today memorable?

Highlights of this Week

1.
2.
3.
4.
5.

Reminder From Your Past Self

Top Priorities For Next Week

1.
2.
3.
4.
5.
6.

Weekly Summary (good/bad/other/weight/etc.)

Workout Summary & Diet Notes:

Sleep Hours

Daily Successes:

1.
2.
3.

TODAY'S GOALS

1.
2.
3.
4.

DONE?

○
○
○
○

Workout Summary & Diet Notes:

Sleep Hours

Daily Successes:

1.
2.
3.

TODAY'S GOALS

1.
2.
3.
4.

DONE?

○
○
○
○

Workout Summary & Diet Notes:

Sleep Hours

Daily Successes:

1.
2.
3.

TODAY'S GOALS

1.
2.
3.
4.

DONE?

○
○
○
○

Fitness Highlights of this Week

1.
2.
3.
4.
5.

Weekly Fitness Notes

RHR

BP

Total Distance (in miles)

Week

Year

Weight

WEEK 26

WEEK 27

Date: _____

MONDAY

Day in review - What made today memorable?

TUESDAY

Day in review - What made today memorable?

WEDNESDAY

Day in review - What made today memorable?

THURSDAY

Day in review - What made today memorable?

"Follow effective actions with quiet reflection. From the quiet reflection will come even more effective action." — *Peter Drucker*

Workout Summary & Diet Notes:	**TODAY'S GOALS**	**DONE?**
Sleep Hours **Daily Successes:** 1. 2. 3.	1. 2. 3. 4.	○ ○ ○ ○

Workout Summary & Diet Notes:	**TODAY'S GOALS**	**DONE?**
Sleep Hours **Daily Successes:** 1. 2. 3.	1. 2. 3. 4.	○ ○ ○ ○

Workout Summary & Diet Notes:	**TODAY'S GOALS**	**DONE?**
Sleep Hours **Daily Successes:** 1. 2. 3.	1. 2. 3. 4.	○ ○ ○ ○

Workout Summary & Diet Notes:	**TODAY'S GOALS**	**DONE?**
Sleep Hours **Daily Successes:** 1. 2. 3.	1. 2. 3. 4.	○ ○ ○ ○

FRIDAY

Day in review – What made today memorable?

SATURDAY

Day in review – What made today memorable?

SUNDAY

Day in review – What made today memorable?

Highlights of this Week

1.
2.
3.
4.
5.

Reminder From Your Past Self

Top Priorities For Next Week

1.   4.
2.   5.
3.   6.

Weekly Summary (good/bad/other/weight/etc.)

Workout Summary & Diet Notes:	TODAY'S GOALS	DONE?
Sleep Hours	1. _____	◯
	2. _____	◯
Daily Successes:	3. _____	◯
1. _____	4. _____	◯
2. _____		
3. _____		

Workout Summary & Diet Notes:	TODAY'S GOALS	DONE?
Sleep Hours	1. _____	◯
	2. _____	◯
Daily Successes:	3. _____	◯
1. _____	4. _____	◯
2. _____		
3. _____		

Workout Summary & Diet Notes:	TODAY'S GOALS	DONE?
Sleep Hours	1. _____	◯
	2. _____	◯
Daily Successes:	3. _____	◯
1. _____	4. _____	◯
2. _____		
3. _____		

Fitness Highlights of this Week

1. _____
2. _____
3. _____
4. _____
5. _____

Weekly Fitness Notes

RHR

BP

Total Distance (in miles)

Week [ ] Year [ ]

Weight [ ]

WEEK 27

WEEK 28

Date: _____

MONDAY

Day in review - What made today memorable?

TUESDAY

Day in review - What made today memorable?

WEDNESDAY

Day in review - What made today memorable?

THURSDAY

Day in review - What made today memorable?

> "If you are not willing to risk the usual, you will have to settle for the ordinary." — *Jim Rohn*

Workout Summary & Diet Notes:	TODAY'S GOALS	DONE?
Sleep Hours	1.	○
	2.	○
Daily Successes:	3.	○
1.		
2.	4.	○
3.		

Workout Summary & Diet Notes:	TODAY'S GOALS	DONE?
Sleep Hours	1.	○
	2.	○
Daily Successes:	3.	○
1.		
2.	4.	○
3.		

Workout Summary & Diet Notes:	TODAY'S GOALS	DONE?
Sleep Hours	1.	○
	2.	○
Daily Successes:	3.	○
1.		
2.	4.	○
3.		

Workout Summary & Diet Notes:	TODAY'S GOALS	DONE?
Sleep Hours	1.	○
	2.	○
Daily Successes:	3.	○
1.		
2.	4.	○
3.		

FRIDAY

Day in review - What made today memorable?

SATURDAY

Day in review - What made today memorable?

SUNDAY

Day in review - What made today memorable?

Highlights of this Week

1. _____
2. _____
3. _____
4. _____
5. _____

Reminder From Your Past Self

Top Priorities For Next Week

1. _____ 4. _____
2. _____ 5. _____
3. _____ 6. _____

Weekly Summary (good/bad/other/weight/etc.)

Workout Summary & Diet Notes:

Sleep Hours

Daily Successes:

1.
2.
3.

TODAY'S GOALS

DONE?

1.
2.
3.
4.

○ ○ ○ ○

Workout Summary & Diet Notes:

Sleep Hours

Daily Successes:

1.
2.
3.

TODAY'S GOALS

DONE?

1.
2.
3.
4.

○ ○ ○ ○

Workout Summary & Diet Notes:

Sleep Hours

Daily Successes:

1.
2.
3.

TODAY'S GOALS

DONE?

1.
2.
3.
4.

○ ○ ○ ○

Fitness Highlights of this Week

1.
2.
3.
4.
5.

Weekly Fitness Notes

RHR

BP

Total Distance (in miles)

Week ____ Year ____

Weight ____

WEEK 28

WEEK 29

Date: _____

MONDAY
Day in review - What made today memorable?

TUESDAY
Day in review - What made today memorable?

WEDNESDAY
Day in review - What made today memorable?

THURSDAY
Day in review - What made today memorable?

> "All progress takes place outside the comfort zone." — *Michael John Bobak*

Workout Summary & Diet Notes:	TODAY'S GOALS	DONE?
Sleep Hours	1. _____	◯
	2. _____	◯
Daily Successes:	3. _____	◯
1. _____	4. _____	◯
2. _____		
3. _____		

Workout Summary & Diet Notes:	TODAY'S GOALS	DONE?
Sleep Hours	1. _____	◯
	2. _____	◯
Daily Successes:	3. _____	◯
1. _____	4. _____	◯
2. _____		
3. _____		

Workout Summary & Diet Notes:	TODAY'S GOALS	DONE?
Sleep Hours	1. _____	◯
	2. _____	◯
Daily Successes:	3. _____	◯
1. _____	4. _____	◯
2. _____		
3. _____		

Workout Summary & Diet Notes:	TODAY'S GOALS	DONE?
Sleep Hours	1. _____	◯
	2. _____	◯
Daily Successes:	3. _____	◯
1. _____	4. _____	◯
2. _____		
3. _____		

FRIDAY

Day in review - What made today memorable?

SATURDAY

Day in review - What made today memorable?

SUNDAY

Day in review - What made today memorable?

Highlights of this Week

1.
2.
3.
4.
5.

Reminder From Your Past Self

Top Priorities For Next Week

1.   4.
2.   5.
3.   6.

Weekly Summary (good/bad/other/weight/etc.)

Workout Summary & Diet Notes:

Sleep Hours

Daily Successes:

1.
2.
3.

TODAY'S GOALS

DONE?

1.
2.
3.
4.

○
○
○
○

Workout Summary & Diet Notes:

Sleep Hours

Daily Successes:

1.
2.
3.

TODAY'S GOALS

DONE?

1.
2.
3.
4.

○
○
○
○

Workout Summary & Diet Notes:

Sleep Hours

Daily Successes:

1.
2.
3.

TODAY'S GOALS

DONE?

1.
2.
3.
4.

○
○
○
○

Fitness Highlights of this Week

1.
2.
3.
4.
5.

Weekly Fitness Notes

RHR

BP

Total Distance
(in miles)

Week | Year

Weight

WEEK 29

How to Win Friends and Influence People

A quick background on this book. It was early 1999, I was 22, had just moved to New York City from Massachusetts for a big career opportunity. One of the first orders of business my company wanted me to do was enroll in Dale Carnegie training for presentation and public speaking practice, as that was going to be a frequent part of my new job.

During the first night of class we were all given this book as part of the course materials and I was hooked immediately. Long before emotional intelligence was a concept that had a name, Dale Carnegie wrote this book which is packed full of practical tips and advice that will easily give you added perspective on your interaction with family, friends, coworkers and virtually anybody else you happen to engage in a conversation with.

This book has sold over 30 million copies since it was published in 1936 and it's entirely possible one of those copies is already in your possession. If that's the case, I would suggest you dust it off and give it a re-read . . . I know I have done that multiple times over the last 20-plus years and I always manage to pick up something new. That's probably the reason it's considered to be a timeless classic for life and business and one that easily stands the test of being just as relevant now as it was over 80 years ago.

Date: _____

MONDAY

Day in review - What made today memorable?

TUESDAY

Day in review - What made today memorable?

WEDNESDAY

Day in review - What made today memorable?

THURSDAY

Day in review - What made today memorable?

> "People who succeed have momentum. The more they succeed, the more they want to succeed, and the more they find a way to succeed. Similarly, when someone is failing, the tendency is to get on a downward spiral that can even become a self-fulfilling prophecy." — *Tony Robbins*

Workout Summary & Diet Notes:	TODAY'S GOALS	DONE?
Sleep Hours **Daily Successes:** 1. 2. 3.	1. 2. 3. 4.	○ ○ ○ ○

Workout Summary & Diet Notes:	TODAY'S GOALS	DONE?
Sleep Hours **Daily Successes:** 1. 2. 3.	1. 2. 3. 4.	○ ○ ○ ○

Workout Summary & Diet Notes:	TODAY'S GOALS	DONE?
Sleep Hours **Daily Successes:** 1. 2. 3.	1. 2. 3. 4.	○ ○ ○ ○

Workout Summary & Diet Notes:	TODAY'S GOALS	DONE?
Sleep Hours **Daily Successes:** 1. 2. 3.	1. 2. 3. 4.	○ ○ ○ ○

FRIDAY

Day in review - What made today memorable?

SATURDAY

Day in review - What made today memorable?

SUNDAY

Day in review - What made today memorable?

Highlights of this Week

1. _____
2. _____
3. _____
4. _____
5. _____

Top Priorities For Next Week

1. _____   4. _____
2. _____   5. _____
3. _____   6. _____

Weekly Summary (good/bad/other/weight/etc.)

Reminder From Your Past Self

Workout Summary & Diet Notes:

Sleep Hours

Daily Successes:

1. _____
2. _____
3. _____

TODAY'S GOALS

DONE?

1. _____ ◯
2. _____ ◯
3. _____ ◯
4. _____ ◯

Workout Summary & Diet Notes:

Sleep Hours

Daily Successes:

1. _____
2. _____
3. _____

TODAY'S GOALS

DONE?

1. _____ ◯
2. _____ ◯
3. _____ ◯
4. _____ ◯

Workout Summary & Diet Notes:

Sleep Hours

Daily Successes:

1. _____
2. _____
3. _____

TODAY'S GOALS

DONE?

1. _____ ◯
2. _____ ◯
3. _____ ◯
4. _____ ◯

Fitness Highlights of this Week

1. _____
2. _____
3. _____
4. _____
5. _____

Weekly Fitness Notes

RHR

BP

Total Distance
(in miles)

Week ☐ Year ☐

Weight
☐

WEEK 30

WEEK 31

Date: _____

MONDAY
Day in review - What made today memorable?

TUESDAY
Day in review - What made today memorable?

WEDNESDAY
Day in review - What made today memorable?

THURSDAY
Day in review - What made today memorable?

"The only limit to our realization of tomorrow will be our doubts of today."
— *Franklin D. Roosevelt*

Workout Summary & Diet Notes:	TODAY'S GOALS	DONE?
Sleep Hours	1. _____	◯
	2. _____	◯
Daily Successes:	3. _____	◯
1. _____	4. _____	◯
2. _____		
3. _____		

Workout Summary & Diet Notes:	TODAY'S GOALS	DONE?
Sleep Hours	1. _____	◯
	2. _____	◯
Daily Successes:	3. _____	◯
1. _____	4. _____	◯
2. _____		
3. _____		

Workout Summary & Diet Notes:	TODAY'S GOALS	DONE?
Sleep Hours	1. _____	◯
	2. _____	◯
Daily Successes:	3. _____	◯
1. _____	4. _____	◯
2. _____		
3. _____		

Workout Summary & Diet Notes:	TODAY'S GOALS	DONE?
Sleep Hours	1. _____	◯
	2. _____	◯
Daily Successes:	3. _____	◯
1. _____	4. _____	◯
2. _____		
3. _____		

FRIDAY

Day in review - What made today memorable?

SATURDAY

Day in review - What made today memorable?

SUNDAY

Day in review - What made today memorable?

Highlights of this Week

1. _____
2. _____
3. _____
4. _____
5. _____

Reminder From Your Past Self

Top Priorities For Next Week

1. _____ 4. _____
2. _____ 5. _____
3. _____ 6. _____

Weekly Summary (good/bad/other/weight/etc.)

Workout Summary & Diet Notes:

Daily Successes:

1. _____
2. _____
3. _____

TODAY'S GOALS

1. _____
2. _____
3. _____
4. _____

DONE?

○
○
○
○

Workout Summary & Diet Notes:

Daily Successes:

1. _____
2. _____
3. _____

TODAY'S GOALS

1. _____
2. _____
3. _____
4. _____

DONE?

○
○
○
○

Workout Summary & Diet Notes:

Daily Successes:

1. _____
2. _____
3. _____

TODAY'S GOALS

1. _____
2. _____
3. _____
4. _____

DONE?

○
○
○
○

Fitness Highlights of this Week

1. _____
2. _____
3. _____
4. _____
5. _____

Weekly Fitness Notes

RHR

BP

Total Distance
(in miles)

Week [ ]   Year [ ]

Weight
[ ]

WEEK 31

WEEK 32

Date: _____

MONDAY

Day in review - What made today memorable?

TUESDAY

Day in review - What made today memorable?

WEDNESDAY

Day in review - What made today memorable?

THURSDAY

Day in review - What made today memorable?

"The way to get started is to quit talking and begin doing." — *Walt Disney*

Workout Summary & Diet Notes:	**TODAY'S GOALS**	**DONE?**
Sleep Hours	1.	○
	2.	○
Daily Successes:	3.	○
1.	4.	○
2.		
3.		

Workout Summary & Diet Notes:	**TODAY'S GOALS**	**DONE?**
Sleep Hours	1.	○
	2.	○
Daily Successes:	3.	○
1.	4.	○
2.		
3.		

Workout Summary & Diet Notes:	**TODAY'S GOALS**	**DONE?**
Sleep Hours	1.	○
	2.	○
Daily Successes:	3.	○
1.	4.	○
2.		
3.		

Workout Summary & Diet Notes:	**TODAY'S GOALS**	**DONE?**
Sleep Hours	1.	○
	2.	○
Daily Successes:	3.	○
1.	4.	○
2.		
3.		

FRIDAY

Day in review - What made today memorable?

SATURDAY

Day in review - What made today memorable?

SUNDAY

Day in review - What made today memorable?

Highlights of this Week

1.
2.
3.
4.
5.

Top Priorities For Next Week

1.   4.
2.   5.
3.   6.

Weekly Summary (good/bad/other/weight/etc.)

Reminder From Your Past Self

Workout Summary & Diet Notes:

Sleep Hours

Daily Successes:
1. _____
2. _____
3. _____

TODAY'S GOALS

1. _____
2. _____
3. _____
4. _____

DONE?

◯
◯
◯
◯

Workout Summary & Diet Notes:

Sleep Hours

Daily Successes:
1. _____
2. _____
3. _____

TODAY'S GOALS

1. _____
2. _____
3. _____
4. _____

DONE?

◯
◯
◯
◯

Workout Summary & Diet Notes:

Sleep Hours

Daily Successes:
1. _____
2. _____
3. _____

TODAY'S GOALS

1. _____
2. _____
3. _____
4. _____

DONE?

◯
◯
◯
◯

Fitness Highlights of this Week

1. _____
2. _____
3. _____
4. _____
5. _____

Weekly Fitness Notes

RHR

BP

Total Distance (in miles)

Week [ ] Year [ ]

Weight [ ]

WEEK 32

WEEK 33

Date: _____

MONDAY

Day in review - What made today memorable?

TUESDAY

Day in review - What made today memorable?

WEDNESDAY

Day in review - What made today memorable?

THURSDAY

Day in review - What made today memorable?

"The successful warrior is the average man, with laser-like focus."
— *Bruce Lee*

Workout Summary & Diet Notes:	TODAY'S GOALS	DONE?
Sleep Hours	1.	◯
	2.	◯
Daily Successes:	3.	◯
1.	4.	◯
2.		
3.		

Workout Summary & Diet Notes:	TODAY'S GOALS	DONE?
Sleep Hours	1.	◯
	2.	◯
Daily Successes:	3.	◯
1.	4.	◯
2.		
3.		

Workout Summary & Diet Notes:	TODAY'S GOALS	DONE?
Sleep Hours	1.	◯
	2.	◯
Daily Successes:	3.	◯
1.	4.	◯
2.		
3.		

Workout Summary & Diet Notes:	TODAY'S GOALS	DONE?
Sleep Hours	1.	◯
	2.	◯
Daily Successes:	3.	◯
1.	4.	◯
2.		
3.		

FRIDAY

Day in review - What made today memorable?

SATURDAY

Day in review - What made today memorable?

SUNDAY

Day in review - What made today memorable?

Highlights of this Week

1. _____
2. _____
3. _____
4. _____
5. _____

Reminder From Your Past Self

Top Priorities For Next Week

1. _____   4. _____
2. _____   5. _____
3. _____   6. _____

Weekly Summary (good/bad/other/weight/etc.)

Workout Summary & Diet Notes:

Sleep Hours

Daily Successes:

1.
2.
3.

TODAY'S GOALS

DONE?

1.
2.
3.
4.

○
○
○
○

Workout Summary & Diet Notes:

Sleep Hours

Daily Successes:

1.
2.
3.

TODAY'S GOALS

DONE?

1.
2.
3.
4.

○
○
○
○

Workout Summary & Diet Notes:

Sleep Hours

Daily Successes:

1.
2.
3.

TODAY'S GOALS

DONE?

1.
2.
3.
4.

○
○
○
○

Fitness Highlights of this Week

1.
2.
3.
4.
5.

Weekly Fitness Notes

RHR

BP

Total Distance (in miles)

Week

Year

Weight

WEEK 33

The Way of the Seal

This book is one of my definite favorites on the list and I hope you find it as beneficial and applicable to your life as I have. Based on the fact that anybody I have recommended this book to over the years ends up raving about it and also recommending it to others is a good sign!

Primarily this is a book about mindset and mental training to achieve greater levels of success in all areas of your life. A big difference in this book and other options that are out there dealing with mindfulness is that Mark Divine is a retired Navy SEAL Commander and has written a book that reflects his background: no nonsense, results-oriented and heavy on the training.

There are eight principles in the book that cover everything from refining your focus, establishing priorities, building the "Three D's" (discipline, drive and determination), and aspects of mental toughness like controlling attention and response as well as developing emotional resilience. Each "Principle" section is accompanied by exercises . . . the mental equivalent of drop and give me 50!

WEEK 34

Date: _____

MONDAY

Day in review - What made today memorable?

TUESDAY

Day in review - What made today memorable?

WEDNESDAY

Day in review - What made today memorable?

THURSDAY

Day in review - What made today memorable?

"Some people dream of success while others wake up and work."
— *Unknown*

Workout Summary & Diet Notes:	TODAY'S GOALS	DONE?
Sleep Hours **Daily Successes:** 1. _____ 2. _____ 3. _____	1. _____ 2. _____ 3. _____ 4. _____	○ ○ ○ ○
Workout Summary & Diet Notes:	TODAY'S GOALS	DONE?
Sleep Hours **Daily Successes:** 1. _____ 2. _____ 3. _____	1. _____ 2. _____ 3. _____ 4. _____	○ ○ ○ ○
Workout Summary & Diet Notes:	TODAY'S GOALS	DONE?
Sleep Hours **Daily Successes:** 1. _____ 2. _____ 3. _____	1. _____ 2. _____ 3. _____ 4. _____	○ ○ ○ ○
Workout Summary & Diet Notes:	TODAY'S GOALS	DONE?
Sleep Hours **Daily Successes:** 1. _____ 2. _____ 3. _____	1. _____ 2. _____ 3. _____ 4. _____	○ ○ ○ ○

FRIDAY

Day in review - What made today memorable?

SATURDAY

Day in review - What made today memorable?

SUNDAY

Day in review - What made today memorable?

Highlights of this Week

1.
2.
3.
4.
5.

Reminder From Your Past Self

Top Priorities For Next Week

1.   4.
2.   5.
3.   6.

Weekly Summary (good/bad/other/weight/etc.)

Workout Summary & Diet Notes:

Sleep Hours

Daily Successes:
1.
2.
3.

TODAY'S GOALS

DONE?

1.
2.
3.
4.

○ ○ ○ ○

Workout Summary & Diet Notes:

Sleep Hours

Daily Successes:
1.
2.
3.

TODAY'S GOALS

DONE?

1.
2.
3.
4.

○ ○ ○ ○

Workout Summary & Diet Notes:

Sleep Hours

Daily Successes:
1.
2.
3.

TODAY'S GOALS

DONE?

1.
2.
3.
4.

○ ○ ○ ○

Fitness Highlights of this Week

1.
2.
3.
4.
5.

Weekly Fitness Notes

RHR

BP

Total Distance (in miles)

Week

Year

Weight

WEEK 34

WEEK 35

Date: _____

MONDAY
Day in review - What made today memorable?

TUESDAY
Day in review - What made today memorable?

WEDNESDAY
Day in review - What made today memorable?

THURSDAY
Day in review - What made today memorable?

"Amateurs sit and wait for inspiration, the rest of us just get up and go to work." — *Stephen King*

Workout Summary & Diet Notes:	TODAY'S GOALS	DONE?
Sleep Hours **Daily Successes:** 1. 2. 3.	1. 2. 3. 4.	◯ ◯ ◯ ◯
Workout Summary & Diet Notes:	TODAY'S GOALS	DONE?
Sleep Hours **Daily Successes:** 1. 2. 3.	1. 2. 3. 4.	◯ ◯ ◯ ◯
Workout Summary & Diet Notes:	TODAY'S GOALS	DONE?
Sleep Hours **Daily Successes:** 1. 2. 3.	1. 2. 3. 4.	◯ ◯ ◯ ◯
Workout Summary & Diet Notes:	TODAY'S GOALS	DONE?
Sleep Hours **Daily Successes:** 1. 2. 3.	1. 2. 3. 4.	◯ ◯ ◯ ◯

FRIDAY

Day in review – What made today memorable?

SATURDAY

Day in review – What made today memorable?

SUNDAY

Day in review – What made today memorable?

Highlights of this Week

1.
2.
3.
4.
5.

Reminder From Your Past Self

Top Priorities For Next Week

1.   4.
2.   5.
3.   6.

Weekly Summary (good/bad/other/weight/etc.)

Workout Summary & Diet Notes:

Sleep Hours

Daily Successes:

1.
2.
3.

TODAY'S GOALS

1.
2.
3.
4.

DONE?

○
○
○
○

Workout Summary & Diet Notes:

Sleep Hours

Daily Successes:

1.
2.
3.

TODAY'S GOALS

1.
2.
3.
4.

DONE?

○
○
○
○

Workout Summary & Diet Notes:

Sleep Hours

Daily Successes:

1.
2.
3.

TODAY'S GOALS

1.
2.
3.
4.

DONE?

○
○
○
○

Fitness Highlights of this Week

1.
2.
3.
4.
5.

Weekly Fitness Notes

RHR

BP

Total Distance
(in miles)

Week

Year

Weight

WEEK 35

WEEK 36

Date: _____

MONDAY

Day in review - What made today memorable?

TUESDAY

Day in review - What made today memorable?

WEDNESDAY

Day in review - What made today memorable?

THURSDAY

Day in review - What made today memorable?

"Spend eighty percent of your time focusing on the opportunities of tomorrow rather than the problems of yesterday." — *Brian Tracy*

Workout Summary & Diet Notes:	TODAY'S GOALS	DONE?
Sleep Hours	1.	○
	2.	○
Daily Successes:	3.	○
1.		
2.	4.	○
3.		

Workout Summary & Diet Notes:	TODAY'S GOALS	DONE?
Sleep Hours	1.	○
	2.	○
Daily Successes:	3.	○
1.		
2.	4.	○
3.		

Workout Summary & Diet Notes:	TODAY'S GOALS	DONE?
Sleep Hours	1.	○
	2.	○
Daily Successes:	3.	○
1.		
2.	4.	○
3.		

Workout Summary & Diet Notes:	TODAY'S GOALS	DONE?
Sleep Hours	1.	○
	2.	○
Daily Successes:	3.	○
1.		
2.	4.	○
3.		

FRIDAY

Day in review - What made today memorable?

SATURDAY

Day in review - What made today memorable?

SUNDAY

Day in review - What made today memorable?

Highlights of this Week

1.
2.
3.
4.
5.

Reminder From Your Past Self

Top Priorities For Next Week

1.   4.
2.   5.
3.   6.

Weekly Summary (good/bad/other/weight/etc.)

Workout Summary & Diet Notes:

Sleep Hours

Daily Successes:

1. _____
2. _____
3. _____

TODAY'S GOALS

DONE?

1. _____ ◯
2. _____ ◯
3. _____ ◯
4. _____ ◯

Workout Summary & Diet Notes:

Sleep Hours

Daily Successes:

1. _____
2. _____
3. _____

TODAY'S GOALS

DONE?

1. _____ ◯
2. _____ ◯
3. _____ ◯
4. _____ ◯

Workout Summary & Diet Notes:

Sleep Hours

Daily Successes:

1. _____
2. _____
3. _____

TODAY'S GOALS

DONE?

1. _____ ◯
2. _____ ◯
3. _____ ◯
4. _____ ◯

Fitness Highlights of this Week

1. _____
2. _____
3. _____
4. _____
5. _____

Weekly Fitness Notes

RHR

BP

Total Distance (in miles)

Week ____ Year ____

Weight ____

WEEK 36

WEEK 37

Date: _____

MONDAY

Day in review - What made today memorable?

TUESDAY

Day in review - What made today memorable?

WEDNESDAY

Day in review - What made today memorable?

THURSDAY

Day in review - What made today memorable?

"Success is liking yourself, liking what you do, and liking how you do it."
— Maya Angelou

Workout Summary & Diet Notes:	TODAY'S GOALS	DONE?
Sleep Hours	1. _____	◯
	2. _____	◯
Daily Successes:	3. _____	◯
1. _____	4. _____	◯
2. _____		
3. _____		

Workout Summary & Diet Notes:	TODAY'S GOALS	DONE?
Sleep Hours	1. _____	◯
	2. _____	◯
Daily Successes:	3. _____	◯
1. _____	4. _____	◯
2. _____		
3. _____		

Workout Summary & Diet Notes:	TODAY'S GOALS	DONE?
Sleep Hours	1. _____	◯
	2. _____	◯
Daily Successes:	3. _____	◯
1. _____	4. _____	◯
2. _____		
3. _____		

Workout Summary & Diet Notes:	TODAY'S GOALS	DONE?
Sleep Hours	1. _____	◯
	2. _____	◯
Daily Successes:	3. _____	◯
1. _____	4. _____	◯
2. _____		
3. _____		

FRIDAY

Day in review - What made today memorable?

SATURDAY

Day in review - What made today memorable?

SUNDAY

Day in review - What made today memorable?

Highlights of this Week

1.
2.
3.
4.
5.

Reminder From Your Past Self

Top Priorities For Next Week

1.   4.
2.   5.
3.   6.

Weekly Summary (good/bad/other/weight/etc.)

Workout Summary & Diet Notes:

Sleep Hours

Daily Successes:

1.
2.
3.

TODAY'S GOALS

1.
2.
3.
4.

DONE?

○
○
○
○

Workout Summary & Diet Notes:

Sleep Hours

Daily Successes:

1.
2.
3.

TODAY'S GOALS

1.
2.
3.
4.

DONE?

○
○
○
○

Workout Summary & Diet Notes:

Sleep Hours

Daily Successes:

1.
2.
3.

TODAY'S GOALS

1.
2.
3.
4.

DONE?

○
○
○
○

Fitness Highlights of this Week

1.
2.
3.
4.
5.

Weekly Fitness Notes

RHR

BP

Total Distance (in miles)

Week

Year

Weight

WEEK 37

How Emotions Are Made

If we agree in concept with the ancient Greeks' words of wisdom to "Know Thyself" is a good plan, then the natural line of questioning that follows is determining what the best way to go about that endeavor is. This topic has generated theories, academic exploration and philosophical debates dating back to when Plato first floated the idea, so it's safe to say that it's been sparking lively debates centuries before any of us were born.

Barrett's research and book is credited by some of the leading minds in the field of neuroscience and behavioral studies as a breakthrough analysis of how our emotions are created and the science behind new insights on how our brain pieces together our feelings to create perceptions which dictate our actions. In applying new discoveries in psychology and neuroscience to decode how our brains construct emotions, *How Emotions Are Made* acts as very readable translation on how we apply these findings in our own career, parenting, and relationships. This book shows not only why our perception becomes our reality but how we can use that knowledge to create the emotional world that our best self would live in.

WEEK 38

Date: _____

MONDAY
Day in review - What made today memorable?

TUESDAY
Day in review - What made today memorable?

WEDNESDAY
Day in review - What made today memorable?

THURSDAY
Day in review - What made today memorable?

"A successful man is one who can lay a firm foundation with the bricks that others throw at him." — *David Brinkley*

Workout Summary & Diet Notes:	TODAY'S GOALS	DONE?
Sleep Hours	1. _____	◯
	2. _____	◯
Daily Successes:	3. _____	◯
1. _____	4. _____	◯
2. _____		
3. _____		

Workout Summary & Diet Notes:	TODAY'S GOALS	DONE?
Sleep Hours	1. _____	◯
	2. _____	◯
Daily Successes:	3. _____	◯
1. _____	4. _____	◯
2. _____		
3. _____		

Workout Summary & Diet Notes:	TODAY'S GOALS	DONE?
Sleep Hours	1. _____	◯
	2. _____	◯
Daily Successes:	3. _____	◯
1. _____	4. _____	◯
2. _____		
3. _____		

Workout Summary & Diet Notes:	TODAY'S GOALS	DONE?
Sleep Hours	1. _____	◯
	2. _____	◯
Daily Successes:	3. _____	◯
1. _____	4. _____	◯
2. _____		
3. _____		

FRIDAY

Day in review - What made today memorable?

SATURDAY

Day in review - What made today memorable?

SUNDAY

Day in review - What made today memorable?

Highlights of this Week

1.
2.
3.
4.
5.

Reminder From Your Past Self

Top Priorities For Next Week

1.   4.
2.   5.
3.   6.

Weekly Summary (good/bad/other/weight/etc.)

Workout Summary & Diet Notes:

Sleep Hours

Daily Successes:

1.
2.
3.

TODAY'S GOALS

1.
2.
3.
4.

DONE?

○
○
○
○

Workout Summary & Diet Notes:

Sleep Hours

Daily Successes:

1.
2.
3.

TODAY'S GOALS

1.
2.
3.
4.

DONE?

○
○
○
○

Workout Summary & Diet Notes:

Sleep Hours

Daily Successes:

1.
2.
3.

TODAY'S GOALS

1.
2.
3.
4.

DONE?

○
○
○
○

Fitness Highlights of this Week

1.
2.
3.
4.
5.

Weekly Fitness Notes

RHR

BP

Total Distance (in miles)

Week

Year

Weight

WEEK 38

WEEK 39

Date: _____

MONDAY

Day in review - What made today memorable?

TUESDAY

Day in review - What made today memorable?

WEDNESDAY

Day in review - What made today memorable?

THURSDAY

Day in review - What made today memorable?

"Don't be distracted by criticism. Remember—the only taste of success some people get is to take a bite out of you." — *Zig Ziglar*

Workout Summary & Diet Notes:

Sleep Hours

Daily Successes:

1. _____
2. _____
3. _____

TODAY'S GOALS

1. _____
2. _____
3. _____
4. _____

DONE?

○
○
○
○

Workout Summary & Diet Notes:

Sleep Hours

Daily Successes:

1. _____
2. _____
3. _____

TODAY'S GOALS

1. _____
2. _____
3. _____
4. _____

DONE?

○
○
○
○

Workout Summary & Diet Notes:

Sleep Hours

Daily Successes:

1. _____
2. _____
3. _____

TODAY'S GOALS

1. _____
2. _____
3. _____
4. _____

DONE?

○
○
○
○

Workout Summary & Diet Notes:

Sleep Hours

Daily Successes:

1. _____
2. _____
3. _____

TODAY'S GOALS

1. _____
2. _____
3. _____
4. _____

DONE?

○
○
○
○

FRIDAY

Day in review - What made today memorable?

SATURDAY

Day in review - What made today memorable?

SUNDAY

Day in review - What made today memorable?

Highlights of this Week

1.
2.
3.
4.
5.

Top Priorities For Next Week

1.   4.
2.   5.
3.   6.

Weekly Summary (good/bad/other/weight/etc.)

Reminder From Your Past Self

Workout Summary & Diet Notes:

Sleep Hours

Daily Successes:

1.
2.
3.

TODAY'S GOALS

DONE?

1.
2.
3.
4.

○
○
○
○

Workout Summary & Diet Notes:

Sleep Hours

Daily Successes:

1.
2.
3.

TODAY'S GOALS

DONE?

1.
2.
3.
4.

○
○
○
○

Workout Summary & Diet Notes:

Sleep Hours

Daily Successes:

1.
2.
3.

TODAY'S GOALS

DONE?

1.
2.
3.
4.

○
○
○
○

Fitness Highlights of this Week

1.
2.
3.
4.
5.

Weekly Fitness Notes

RHR

BP

Total Distance
(in miles)

Week

Year

Weight

WEEK 39

WEEK 40

Date: _____

MONDAY
Day in review - What made today memorable?

TUESDAY
Day in review - What made today memorable?

WEDNESDAY
Day in review - What made today memorable?

THURSDAY
Day in review - What made today memorable?

"The secret of success is to do the common thing uncommonly well."
— *John D. Rockefeller*

Workout Summary & Diet Notes:	TODAY'S GOALS	DONE?
Sleep Hours **Daily Successes:** 1. 2. 3.	1. 2. 3. 4.	○ ○ ○ ○

Workout Summary & Diet Notes:	TODAY'S GOALS	DONE?
Sleep Hours **Daily Successes:** 1. 2. 3.	1. 2. 3. 4.	○ ○ ○ ○

Workout Summary & Diet Notes:	TODAY'S GOALS	DONE?
Sleep Hours **Daily Successes:** 1. 2. 3.	1. 2. 3. 4.	○ ○ ○ ○

Workout Summary & Diet Notes:	TODAY'S GOALS	DONE?
Sleep Hours **Daily Successes:** 1. 2. 3.	1. 2. 3. 4.	○ ○ ○ ○

FRIDAY

Day in review - What made today memorable?

SATURDAY

Day in review - What made today memorable?

SUNDAY

Day in review - What made today memorable?

Highlights of this Week

1.
2.
3.
4.
5.

Reminder From Your Past Self

Top Priorities For Next Week

1.   4.
2.   5.
3.   6.

Weekly Summary (good/bad/other/weight/etc.)

Workout Summary & Diet Notes:

Sleep Hours

Daily Successes:

1.
2.
3.

TODAY'S GOALS

1.
2.
3.
4.

DONE?

○
○
○
○

Workout Summary & Diet Notes:

Sleep Hours

Daily Successes:

1.
2.
3.

TODAY'S GOALS

1.
2.
3.
4.

DONE?

○
○
○
○

Workout Summary & Diet Notes:

Sleep Hours

Daily Successes:

1.
2.
3.

TODAY'S GOALS

1.
2.
3.
4.

DONE?

○
○
○
○

Fitness Highlights of this Week

1.
2.
3.
4.
5.

Weekly Fitness Notes

RHR

BP

Total Distance (in miles)

Week ____   Year ____

Weight ____

WEEK 40

WEEK 41

Date: _____

MONDAY

Day in review - What made today memorable?

TUESDAY

Day in review - What made today memorable?

WEDNESDAY

Day in review - What made today memorable?

THURSDAY

Day in review - What made today memorable?

> "Optimism is the most important human trait, because it allows us to evolve our ideas, to improve our situation, and to hope for a better tomorrow."
> — *Seth Godin*

Workout Summary & Diet Notes:	TODAY'S GOALS	DONE?
Sleep Hours	1. _____	◯
	2. _____	◯
Daily Successes:	3. _____	◯
1. _____		
2. _____	4. _____	◯
3. _____		

Workout Summary & Diet Notes:	TODAY'S GOALS	DONE?
Sleep Hours	1. _____	◯
	2. _____	◯
Daily Successes:	3. _____	◯
1. _____		
2. _____	4. _____	◯
3. _____		

Workout Summary & Diet Notes:	TODAY'S GOALS	DONE?
Sleep Hours	1. _____	◯
	2. _____	◯
Daily Successes:	3. _____	◯
1. _____		
2. _____	4. _____	◯
3. _____		

Workout Summary & Diet Notes:	TODAY'S GOALS	DONE?
Sleep Hours	1. _____	◯
	2. _____	◯
Daily Successes:	3. _____	◯
1. _____		
2. _____	4. _____	◯
3. _____		

FRIDAY

Day in review - What made today memorable?

SATURDAY

Day in review - What made today memorable?

SUNDAY

Day in review - What made today memorable?

Highlights of this Week

1.
2.
3.
4.
5.

Reminder From Your Past Self

Top Priorities For Next Week

1.   4.
2.   5.
3.   6.

Weekly Summary (good/bad/other/weight/etc.)

Workout Summary & Diet Notes:

Sleep Hours

Daily Successes:

1.
2.
3.

TODAY'S GOALS

DONE?

1.
2.
3.
4.

○
○
○
○

Workout Summary & Diet Notes:

Sleep Hours

Daily Successes:

1.
2.
3.

TODAY'S GOALS

DONE?

1.
2.
3.
4.

○
○
○
○

Workout Summary & Diet Notes:

Sleep Hours

Daily Successes:

1.
2.
3.

TODAY'S GOALS

DONE?

1.
2.
3.
4.

○
○
○
○

Fitness Highlights of this Week

1.
2.
3.
4.
5.

Weekly Fitness Notes

RHR

BP

Total Distance
(in miles)

Week

Year

Weight

WEEK 41

The 7 Habits of Highly Effective People

I feel that this book and *How to Win Friends and Influence People* are similar selections in the sense that both are titles you are most likely familiar with and possibly have already read. Also, both books are considered game-changing classics and as such, are worthy of a re-read periodically. This reasoning makes it a win-win whether you have or have not already read it which is why I include them on the list. If you have not read *The 7 Habits* book yet you are certainly in for an enlightening month of reading some new ideas and approaches that directly apply to the mindset principles of continuous improvement central to the BAR40 life.

The title is a bit of a simplification in the sense that this book is much more than a list of seven habits. More to the core of the content would be to say the book is a resource on self-mastery and how to become as effective as possible by tapping into our own natural and renewable resources. While *The Power of Habit* starts the year of BAR40 suggested reading, *The 7 Habits* fits in perfectly toward the end of the year in building further on the foundation of implementing these powerful forces of change in our daily life that bring profound effects in all areas.

WEEK 42

Date: _____

MONDAY

Day in review – What made today memorable?

TUESDAY

Day in review – What made today memorable?

WEDNESDAY

Day in review – What made today memorable?

THURSDAY

Day in review – What made today memorable?

Opportunity is missed by most people because it is dressed in overalls and looks like hard work." — *Thomas Edison*

Workout Summary & Diet Notes:	TODAY'S GOALS	DONE?
Sleep Hours	1. _____	○
	2. _____	○
Daily Successes:	3. _____	○
1. _____	4. _____	○
2. _____		
3. _____		

Workout Summary & Diet Notes:	TODAY'S GOALS	DONE?
Sleep Hours	1. _____	○
	2. _____	○
Daily Successes:	3. _____	○
1. _____	4. _____	○
2. _____		
3. _____		

Workout Summary & Diet Notes:	TODAY'S GOALS	DONE?
Sleep Hours	1. _____	○
	2. _____	○
Daily Successes:	3. _____	○
1. _____	4. _____	○
2. _____		
3. _____		

Workout Summary & Diet Notes:	TODAY'S GOALS	DONE?
Sleep Hours	1. _____	○
	2. _____	○
Daily Successes:	3. _____	○
1. _____	4. _____	○
2. _____		
3. _____		

FRIDAY

Day in review - What made today memorable?

SATURDAY

Day in review - What made today memorable?

SUNDAY

Day in review - What made today memorable?

Highlights of this Week

1.
2.
3.
4.
5.

Reminder From Your Past Self

Top Priorities For Next Week

1.   4.
2.   5.
3.   6.

Weekly Summary (good/bad/other/weight/etc.)

Workout Summary & Diet Notes:

Sleep
Hours

Daily Successes:

1.
2.
3.

TODAY'S GOALS

1.
2.
3.
4.

DONE?

○
○
○
○

Workout Summary & Diet Notes:

Sleep
Hours

Daily Successes:

1.
2.
3.

TODAY'S GOALS

1.
2.
3.
4.

DONE?

○
○
○
○

Workout Summary & Diet Notes:

Sleep
Hours

Daily Successes:

1.
2.
3.

TODAY'S GOALS

1.
2.
3.
4.

DONE?

○
○
○
○

Fitness Highlights of this Week

1.
2.
3.
4.
5.

Weekly Fitness Notes

RHR

BP

Total Distance
(in miles)

Week   Year

Weight

WEEK 42

WEEK 43

Date: _____

MONDAY

Day in review - What made today memorable?

TUESDAY

Day in review - What made today memorable?

WEDNESDAY

Day in review - What made today memorable?

THURSDAY

Day in review - What made today memorable?

> "The only place where success comes before work is in the dictionary."
> — *Vidal Sassoon*

Workout Summary & Diet Notes:	TODAY'S GOALS	DONE?
Sleep Hours	1. _____	◯
	2. _____	◯
Daily Successes:	3. _____	◯
1. _____		
2. _____	4. _____	◯
3. _____		

Workout Summary & Diet Notes:	TODAY'S GOALS	DONE?
Sleep Hours	1. _____	◯
	2. _____	◯
Daily Successes:	3. _____	◯
1. _____		
2. _____	4. _____	◯
3. _____		

Workout Summary & Diet Notes:	TODAY'S GOALS	DONE?
Sleep Hours	1. _____	◯
	2. _____	◯
Daily Successes:	3. _____	◯
1. _____		
2. _____	4. _____	◯
3. _____		

Workout Summary & Diet Notes:	TODAY'S GOALS	DONE?
Sleep Hours	1. _____	◯
	2. _____	◯
Daily Successes:	3. _____	◯
1. _____		
2. _____	4. _____	◯
3. _____		

FRIDAY

Day in review – What made today memorable?

SATURDAY

Day in review – What made today memorable?

SUNDAY

Day in review – What made today memorable?

Highlights of this Week

1.
2.
3.
4.
5.

Reminder From Your Past Self

Top Priorities For Next Week

1.   4.
2.   5.
3.   6.

Weekly Summary (good/bad/other/weight/etc.)

Workout Summary & Diet Notes:

Sleep Hours

Daily Successes:

1.
2.
3.

TODAY'S GOALS

DONE?

1.
2.
3.
4.

Workout Summary & Diet Notes:

Sleep Hours

Daily Successes:

1.
2.
3.

TODAY'S GOALS

DONE?

1.
2.
3.
4.

Workout Summary & Diet Notes:

Sleep Hours

Daily Successes:

1.
2.
3.

TODAY'S GOALS

DONE?

1.
2.
3.
4.

Fitness Highlights of this Week

1.
2.
3.
4.
5.

Weekly Fitness Notes

RHR

BP

Total Distance
(in miles)

Week

Year

Weight

WEEK 43

WEEK 44

Date: _____

MONDAY

Day in review - What made today memorable?

TUESDAY

Day in review - What made today memorable?

WEDNESDAY

Day in review - What made today memorable?

THURSDAY

Day in review - What made today memorable?

"To guarantee success, act as if it were impossible to fail."
— *Dorothea Brande*

Workout Summary & Diet Notes:	TODAY'S GOALS	DONE?
Sleep Hours	1. _____	◯
	2. _____	◯
Daily Successes:	3. _____	◯
1. _____		
2. _____	4. _____	◯
3. _____		

Workout Summary & Diet Notes:	TODAY'S GOALS	DONE?
Sleep Hours	1. _____	◯
	2. _____	◯
Daily Successes:	3. _____	◯
1. _____		
2. _____	4. _____	◯
3. _____		

Workout Summary & Diet Notes:	TODAY'S GOALS	DONE?
Sleep Hours	1. _____	◯
	2. _____	◯
Daily Successes:	3. _____	◯
1. _____		
2. _____	4. _____	◯
3. _____		

Workout Summary & Diet Notes:	TODAY'S GOALS	DONE?
Sleep Hours	1. _____	◯
	2. _____	◯
Daily Successes:	3. _____	◯
1. _____		
2. _____	4. _____	◯
3. _____		

FRIDAY

Day in review - What made today memorable?

SATURDAY

Day in review - What made today memorable?

SUNDAY

Day in review - What made today memorable?

Highlights of this Week

1. _____
2. _____
3. _____
4. _____
5. _____

Reminder From Your Past Self

Top Priorities For Next Week

1. _____ 4. _____
2. _____ 5. _____
3. _____ 6. _____

Weekly Summary (good/bad/other/weight/etc.)

Workout Summary & Diet Notes:

Sleep Hours

Daily Successes:

1.
2.
3.

TODAY'S GOALS

1.
2.
3.
4.

DONE?

○
○
○
○

Workout Summary & Diet Notes:

Sleep Hours

Daily Successes:

1.
2.
3.

TODAY'S GOALS

1.
2.
3.
4.

DONE?

○
○
○
○

Workout Summary & Diet Notes:

Sleep Hours

Daily Successes:

1.
2.
3.

TODAY'S GOALS

1.
2.
3.
4.

DONE?

○
○
○
○

Fitness Highlights of this Week

1.
2.
3.
4.
5.

Weekly Fitness Notes

RHR

BP

Total Distance (in miles)

Week

Year

Weight

WEEK 44

WEEK 45

Date: _____

MONDAY

Day in review - What made today memorable?

TUESDAY

Day in review - What made today memorable?

WEDNESDAY

Day in review - What made today memorable?

THURSDAY

Day in review - What made today memorable?

> "Don't judge each day by the harvest you reap but by the seeds that you plant." — *Robert Stevenson*

Workout Summary & Diet Notes:	TODAY'S GOALS	DONE?
Sleep Hours	1. _____	○
	2. _____	○
Daily Successes:	3. _____	○
1. _____	4. _____	○
2. _____		
3. _____		

Workout Summary & Diet Notes:	TODAY'S GOALS	DONE?
Sleep Hours	1. _____	○
	2. _____	○
Daily Successes:	3. _____	○
1. _____	4. _____	○
2. _____		
3. _____		

Workout Summary & Diet Notes:	TODAY'S GOALS	DONE?
Sleep Hours	1. _____	○
	2. _____	○
Daily Successes:	3. _____	○
1. _____	4. _____	○
2. _____		
3. _____		

Workout Summary & Diet Notes:	TODAY'S GOALS	DONE?
Sleep Hours	1. _____	○
	2. _____	○
Daily Successes:	3. _____	○
1. _____	4. _____	○
2. _____		
3. _____		

FRIDAY

Day in review - What made today memorable?

SATURDAY

Day in review - What made today memorable?

SUNDAY

Day in review - What made today memorable?

Highlights of this Week

1.
2.
3.
4.
5.

Top Priorities For Next Week

1.
2.
3.
4.
5.
6.

Weekly Summary (good/bad/other/weight/etc.)

Reminder From Your Past Self

Workout Summary & Diet Notes:

Sleep Hours

Daily Successes:

1.
2.
3.

TODAY'S GOALS

DONE?

1. ◯
2. ◯
3. ◯
4. ◯

Workout Summary & Diet Notes:

Sleep Hours

Daily Successes:

1.
2.
3.

TODAY'S GOALS

DONE?

1. ◯
2. ◯
3. ◯
4. ◯

Workout Summary & Diet Notes:

Sleep Hours

Daily Successes:

1.
2.
3.

TODAY'S GOALS

DONE?

1. ◯
2. ◯
3. ◯
4. ◯

Fitness Highlights of this Week

1.
2.
3.
4.
5.

Weekly Fitness Notes

RHR

BP

Total Distance (in miles)

Week

Year

Weight

WEEK 45

The Slight Edge

I came across this book fairly recently and it hit home in all the areas of the BAR40 philosophy of continuous improvement and personal accountability. I'm confident you will find this to be a useful addition to the 2020 Suggested Reading List as it does a great job of reinforcing a key idea. Fundamentally, the concept of how the daily discipline of making the slightly tougher, but better, choice in all the small things results in a gradual but steady trajectory of success versus the majority of people who live life looking for the quickest and easiest way to do something without much thought to the big picture.

Jeff Olson points out he did not invent or create some radical new solution but instead this book is all about explaining how a simple philosophy applied consistently over time is creating the mindset and path in life that repels failure.

I think you will also find this book useful in considering the power of compounding, in which small efforts yield large results over time. Instead of a financial example of watching $1,000 grow into $1 million from interest growing on interest, it deals with small slightly better choices (hence *The Slight Edge* title) becoming a lifetime of positive results.

WEEK 46

Date: _____

MONDAY

Day in review - What made today memorable?

TUESDAY

Day in review - What made today memorable?

WEDNESDAY

Day in review - What made today memorable?

THURSDAY

Day in review - What made today memorable?

"The question isn't who is going to let me; it's who is going to stop me."
— *Ayn Rand*

Workout Summary & Diet Notes:	TODAY'S GOALS	DONE?
Sleep Hours	1. _____	◯
	2. _____	◯
Daily Successes:	3. _____	◯
1. _____	4. _____	◯
2. _____		
3. _____		

Workout Summary & Diet Notes:	TODAY'S GOALS	DONE?
Sleep Hours	1. _____	◯
	2. _____	◯
Daily Successes:	3. _____	◯
1. _____	4. _____	◯
2. _____		
3. _____		

Workout Summary & Diet Notes:	TODAY'S GOALS	DONE?
Sleep Hours	1. _____	◯
	2. _____	◯
Daily Successes:	3. _____	◯
1. _____	4. _____	◯
2. _____		
3. _____		

Workout Summary & Diet Notes:	TODAY'S GOALS	DONE?
Sleep Hours	1. _____	◯
	2. _____	◯
Daily Successes:	3. _____	◯
1. _____	4. _____	◯
2. _____		
3. _____		

FRIDAY

Day in review - What made today memorable?

SATURDAY

Day in review - What made today memorable?

SUNDAY

Day in review - What made today memorable?

Highlights of this Week

1. _____
2. _____
3. _____
4. _____
5. _____

Top Priorities For Next Week

1. _____ 4. _____
2. _____ 5. _____
3. _____ 6. _____

Weekly Summary (good/bad/other/weight/etc.)

Reminder From Your Past Self

Workout Summary & Diet Notes:

Sleep Hours

Daily Successes:

1.
2.
3.

TODAY'S GOALS

1.
2.
3.
4.

DONE?

○
○
○
○

Workout Summary & Diet Notes:

Sleep Hours

Daily Successes:

1.
2.
3.

TODAY'S GOALS

1.
2.
3.
4.

DONE?

○
○
○
○

Workout Summary & Diet Notes:

Sleep Hours

Daily Successes:

1.
2.
3.

TODAY'S GOALS

1.
2.
3.
4.

DONE?

○
○
○
○

Fitness Highlights of this Week

1.
2.
3.
4.
5.

Weekly Fitness Notes

RHR

BP

Total Distance (in miles)

Week

Year

Weight

WEEK 46

WEEK 47

Date: _____

MONDAY
Day in review - What made today memorable?

TUESDAY
Day in review - What made today memorable?

WEDNESDAY
Day in review - What made today memorable?

THURSDAY
Day in review - What made today memorable?

"Keep away from people who try to belittle your ambitions. Small people always do that, but the really great make you feel that you, too, can become great." — *Mark Twain*

Workout Summary & Diet Notes:	TODAY'S GOALS	DONE?
Sleep Hours	1. _____	◯
	2. _____	◯
Daily Successes:	3. _____	◯
1. _____	4. _____	◯
2. _____		
3. _____		

Workout Summary & Diet Notes:	TODAY'S GOALS	DONE?
Sleep Hours	1. _____	◯
	2. _____	◯
Daily Successes:	3. _____	◯
1. _____	4. _____	◯
2. _____		
3. _____		

Workout Summary & Diet Notes:	TODAY'S GOALS	DONE?
Sleep Hours	1. _____	◯
	2. _____	◯
Daily Successes:	3. _____	◯
1. _____	4. _____	◯
2. _____		
3. _____		

Workout Summary & Diet Notes:	TODAY'S GOALS	DONE?
Sleep Hours	1. _____	◯
	2. _____	◯
Daily Successes:	3. _____	◯
1. _____	4. _____	◯
2. _____		
3. _____		

FRIDAY

Day in review – What made today memorable?

SATURDAY

Day in review – What made today memorable?

SUNDAY

Day in review – What made today memorable?

Highlights of this Week	Top Priorities For Next Week
1. _____	1. _____ 4. _____
2. _____	2. _____ 5. _____
3. _____	3. _____ 6. _____
4. _____	**Weekly Summary** (good/bad/other/weight/etc.)
5. _____	

Reminder From Your Past Self

Workout Summary & Diet Notes:

Sleep Hours

Daily Successes:

1.
2.
3.

TODAY'S GOALS

1.
2.
3.
4.

DONE?

○
○
○
○

Workout Summary & Diet Notes:

Sleep Hours

Daily Successes:

1.
2.
3.

TODAY'S GOALS

1.
2.
3.
4.

DONE?

○
○
○
○

Workout Summary & Diet Notes:

Sleep Hours

Daily Successes:

1.
2.
3.

TODAY'S GOALS

1.
2.
3.
4.

DONE?

○
○
○
○

Fitness Highlights of this Week

1.
2.
3.
4.
5.

Weekly Fitness Notes

RHR

BP

Total Distance (in miles)

Week

Year

Weight

WEEK 47

WEEK 48

Date: _____

MONDAY

Day in review - What made today memorable?

TUESDAY

Day in review - What made today memorable?

WEDNESDAY

Day in review - What made today memorable?

THURSDAY

Day in review - What made today memorable?

> "Live as if you were to die tomorrow. Learn as if you were to live forever."
> — *Mahatma Gandhi*

Workout Summary & Diet Notes:	TODAY'S GOALS	DONE?
Sleep Hours	1. _____	○
	2. _____	○
Daily Successes:	3. _____	○
1. _____		
2. _____	4. _____	○
3. _____		

Workout Summary & Diet Notes:	TODAY'S GOALS	DONE?
Sleep Hours	1. _____	○
	2. _____	○
Daily Successes:	3. _____	○
1. _____		
2. _____	4. _____	○
3. _____		

Workout Summary & Diet Notes:	TODAY'S GOALS	DONE?
Sleep Hours	1. _____	○
	2. _____	○
Daily Successes:	3. _____	○
1. _____		
2. _____	4. _____	○
3. _____		

Workout Summary & Diet Notes:	TODAY'S GOALS	DONE?
Sleep Hours	1. _____	○
	2. _____	○
Daily Successes:	3. _____	○
1. _____		
2. _____	4. _____	○
3. _____		

FRIDAY

Day in review - What made today memorable?

SATURDAY

Day in review - What made today memorable?

SUNDAY

Day in review - What made today memorable?

Highlights of this Week

1.
2.
3.
4.
5.

Reminder From Your Past Self

Top Priorities For Next Week

1.   4.
2.   5.
3.   6.

Weekly Summary (good/bad/other/weight/etc.)

Workout Summary & Diet Notes:	TODAY'S GOALS	DONE?
Sleep Hours	1. _____	◯
	2. _____	◯
Daily Successes:	3. _____	◯
1. _____	4. _____	◯
2. _____		
3. _____		

Workout Summary & Diet Notes:	TODAY'S GOALS	DONE?
Sleep Hours	1. _____	◯
	2. _____	◯
Daily Successes:	3. _____	◯
1. _____	4. _____	◯
2. _____		
3. _____		

Workout Summary & Diet Notes:	TODAY'S GOALS	DONE?
Sleep Hours	1. _____	◯
	2. _____	◯
Daily Successes:	3. _____	◯
1. _____	4. _____	◯
2. _____		
3. _____		

Fitness Highlights of this Week

1. _____
2. _____
3. _____
4. _____
5. _____

Weekly Fitness Notes

RHR

BP

Total Distance (in miles)	Weight	
Week ☐ Year ☐	☐	**WEEK 48**

WEEK 49

Date: _____

MONDAY

Day in review - What made today memorable?

TUESDAY

Day in review - What made today memorable?

WEDNESDAY

Day in review - What made today memorable?

THURSDAY

Day in review - What made today memorable?

"Whenever you see a successful person, you only see the public glories, never the private sacrifices to reach them." — *Vaibhav Shah*

Workout Summary & Diet Notes:	TODAY'S GOALS	DONE?
Sleep Hours	1. _____	◯
	2. _____	◯
Daily Successes:	3. _____	◯
1. _____	4. _____	◯
2. _____		
3. _____		

Workout Summary & Diet Notes:	TODAY'S GOALS	DONE?
Sleep Hours	1. _____	◯
	2. _____	◯
Daily Successes:	3. _____	◯
1. _____	4. _____	◯
2. _____		
3. _____		

Workout Summary & Diet Notes:	TODAY'S GOALS	DONE?
Sleep Hours	1. _____	◯
	2. _____	◯
Daily Successes:	3. _____	◯
1. _____	4. _____	◯
2. _____		
3. _____		

Workout Summary & Diet Notes:	TODAY'S GOALS	DONE?
Sleep Hours	1. _____	◯
	2. _____	◯
Daily Successes:	3. _____	◯
1. _____	4. _____	◯
2. _____		
3. _____		

FRIDAY

Day in review - What made today memorable?

SATURDAY

Day in review - What made today memorable?

SUNDAY

Day in review - What made today memorable?

Highlights of this Week

1. _____
2. _____
3. _____
4. _____
5. _____

Reminder From Your Past Self

Top Priorities For Next Week

1. _____   4. _____
2. _____   5. _____
3. _____   6. _____

Weekly Summary (good/bad/other/weight/etc.)

Workout Summary & Diet Notes:

Sleep Hours

Daily Successes:

1.
2.
3.

TODAY'S GOALS

1.
2.
3.
4.

DONE?

○
○
○
○

Workout Summary & Diet Notes:

Sleep Hours

Daily Successes:

1.
2.
3.

TODAY'S GOALS

1.
2.
3.
4.

DONE?

○
○
○
○

Workout Summary & Diet Notes:

Sleep Hours

Daily Successes:

1.
2.
3.

TODAY'S GOALS

1.
2.
3.
4.

DONE?

○
○
○
○

Fitness Highlights of this Week

1.
2.
3.
4.
5.

Weekly Fitness Notes

RHR

BP

Total Distance (in miles)

Week

Year

Weight

WEEK 49

Alcohol Explained

Similar to the Drinking section in the book, I saved *Alcohol Explained* until the end and for a similar reason. Simply put, you may have chosen to opt out of the 52-week "dry" component of BAR40 and if that's the case, neither that section nor this book may be of any interest to you. If that is the case then by all means feel free to skip it, although I will point out that even if you are not looking to stop drinking (or don't drink currently), *Alcohol Explained* does provide a wealth of information that you may find useful to know in the case there are other people in your life that would benefit from you gaining knowledge on the subject.

That said, in the event you have given up drinking for the 52 weeks, congratulations on a fantastic accomplishment and I hope it was an all-around awesome experience that gave your life an overall boost both physically and mentally. At 49 weeks into an alcohol-free life you will have experienced firsthand the profound benefits that come along with allowing your mind and body to operate free of the mental and physical restraints that drinking brings. Even knowing those benefits, this book will still be something that you will appreciate in that it gives all the reinforcing reasoning behind why we feel so great. Porter does an excellent job of pulling back the curtain on what goes on internally when we drink and how alcohol operates as an addictive substance. If you like the idea of going back to carefree and fun drinking in four weeks when BAR40 is complete, then I give you advance warning that you will not be able to put the toothpaste back in the tube when it comes to how you perceive drinking after reading this book!

It's hard to go on enjoying magic shows after you see a be-hind the scenes documentary of how all the convincing illu-sions are actually done. As expertly as the beer, wine and spirits industry has marketed their products into a romanticized, good-time necessity . . . *Alcohol Explained* dismantles the ideas in a matter-of-fact way by pointing out the how's and why's of how we feel before, during and after drinking. I do think this book would be highly useful for anybody struggling with any sort of "one day at a time" approach as that mindset indicates there is still an urge to drink that is being fought against using sheer willpower. After reading *Alcohol Explained,* whatever desire you had to drink may have left the building! If you find this topic as interesting as I did and you and want to read more about this fascinating mass-marketed toxin, another great book to read is *Alcohol Lied to Me* by Craig Beck.

This brings us to the end of the year's list. Happy reading in your final month of BAR40! I hope you enjoyed the 13 books on the list and considered them to be useful tools in your BAR40 journey. I found each of these books to be very worthwhile reads that all had practical applications in my own life. My intent in suggesting them to you would be that they add similar benefits during your self-guided progression toward your best year ever. I'm very interested in hearing your feedback on them along with any suggestions on additions for the next edition.

WEEK 50

Date: _____

MONDAY

Day in review - What made today memorable?

TUESDAY

Day in review - What made today memorable?

WEDNESDAY

Day in review - What made today memorable?

THURSDAY

Day in review - What made today memorable?

"Self conquest is the greatest of victories." — *Plato*

Workout Summary & Diet Notes:	TODAY'S GOALS	DONE?
Sleep Hours	1. _____	◯
	2. _____	◯
Daily Successes:	3. _____	◯
1. _____	4. _____	◯
2. _____		
3. _____		

Workout Summary & Diet Notes:	TODAY'S GOALS	DONE?
Sleep Hours	1. _____	◯
	2. _____	◯
Daily Successes:	3. _____	◯
1. _____	4. _____	◯
2. _____		
3. _____		

Workout Summary & Diet Notes:	TODAY'S GOALS	DONE?
Sleep Hours	1. _____	◯
	2. _____	◯
Daily Successes:	3. _____	◯
1. _____	4. _____	◯
2. _____		
3. _____		

Workout Summary & Diet Notes:	TODAY'S GOALS	DONE?
Sleep Hours	1. _____	◯
	2. _____	◯
Daily Successes:	3. _____	◯
1. _____	4. _____	◯
2. _____		
3. _____		

FRIDAY

Day in review - What made today memorable?

SATURDAY

Day in review - What made today memorable?

SUNDAY

Day in review - What made today memorable?

Highlights of this Week

1.
2.
3.
4.
5.

Reminder From Your Past Self

Top Priorities For Next Week

1.   4.
2.   5.
3.   6.

Weekly Summary (good/bad/other/weight/etc.)

Workout Summary & Diet Notes:	TODAY'S GOALS	DONE?
Sleep Hours	1. _____	◯
	2. _____	◯
Daily Successes:	3. _____	◯
1. _____	4. _____	◯
2. _____		
3. _____		

Workout Summary & Diet Notes:	TODAY'S GOALS	DONE?
Sleep Hours	1. _____	◯
	2. _____	◯
Daily Successes:	3. _____	◯
1. _____	4. _____	◯
2. _____		
3. _____		

Workout Summary & Diet Notes:	TODAY'S GOALS	DONE?
Sleep Hours	1. _____	◯
	2. _____	◯
Daily Successes:	3. _____	◯
1. _____	4. _____	◯
2. _____		
3. _____		

Fitness Highlights of this Week

1. _____
2. _____
3. _____
4. _____
5. _____

Weekly Fitness Notes

RHR

BP

Total Distance (in miles)

Week [ ] Year [ ]

Weight [ ]

WEEK 50

WEEK 51

Date: _____

MONDAY

Day in review - What made today memorable?

TUESDAY

Day in review - What made today memorable?

WEDNESDAY

Day in review - What made today memorable?

THURSDAY

Day in review - What made today memorable?

> "The best way to predict your future is to create it." — *Peter Drucker*

Workout Summary & Diet Notes:	TODAY'S GOALS	DONE?
Sleep Hours	1. _____	◯
	2. _____	◯
Daily Successes:	3. _____	◯
1. _____		
2. _____	4. _____	◯
3. _____		

Workout Summary & Diet Notes:	TODAY'S GOALS	DONE?
Sleep Hours	1. _____	◯
	2. _____	◯
Daily Successes:	3. _____	◯
1. _____		
2. _____	4. _____	◯
3. _____		

Workout Summary & Diet Notes:	TODAY'S GOALS	DONE?
Sleep Hours	1. _____	◯
	2. _____	◯
Daily Successes:	3. _____	◯
1. _____		
2. _____	4. _____	◯
3. _____		

Workout Summary & Diet Notes:	TODAY'S GOALS	DONE?
Sleep Hours	1. _____	◯
	2. _____	◯
Daily Successes:	3. _____	◯
1. _____		
2. _____	4. _____	◯
3. _____		

FRIDAY

Day in review - What made today memorable?

SATURDAY

Day in review - What made today memorable?

SUNDAY

Day in review - What made today memorable?

Highlights of this Week

1.
2.
3.
4.
5.

Top Priorities For Next Week

1.   4.
2.   5.
3.   6.

Weekly Summary (good/bad/other/weight/etc.)

Reminder From Your Past Self

Workout Summary & Diet Notes:

Sleep
Hours

Daily Successes:

1. _____
2. _____
3. _____

TODAY'S GOALS

1. _____
2. _____
3. _____
4. _____

DONE?

◯
◯
◯
◯

Workout Summary & Diet Notes:

Sleep
Hours

Daily Successes:

1. _____
2. _____
3. _____

TODAY'S GOALS

1. _____
2. _____
3. _____
4. _____

DONE?

◯
◯
◯
◯

Workout Summary & Diet Notes:

Sleep
Hours

Daily Successes:

1. _____
2. _____
3. _____

TODAY'S GOALS

1. _____
2. _____
3. _____
4. _____

DONE?

◯
◯
◯
◯

Fitness Highlights of this Week

1. _____
2. _____
3. _____
4. _____
5. _____

Weekly Fitness Notes

RHR

BP

Total Distance (in miles)

Week [   ]   Year [   ]

Weight

[   ]

WEEK 51

WEEK 52

Date: _____

MONDAY

Day in review - What made today memorable?

TUESDAY

Day in review - What made today memorable?

WEDNESDAY

Day in review - What made today memorable?

THURSDAY

Day in review - What made today memorable?

"Vision without execution is just hallucination" — *Thomas Edison*

Workout Summary & Diet Notes:	TODAY'S GOALS	DONE?
Sleep Hours	1. _____	◯
	2. _____	◯
Daily Successes:	3. _____	◯
1. _____	4. _____	◯
2. _____		
3. _____		

Workout Summary & Diet Notes:	TODAY'S GOALS	DONE?
Sleep Hours	1. _____	◯
	2. _____	◯
Daily Successes:	3. _____	◯
1. _____	4. _____	◯
2. _____		
3. _____		

Workout Summary & Diet Notes:	TODAY'S GOALS	DONE?
Sleep Hours	1. _____	◯
	2. _____	◯
Daily Successes:	3. _____	◯
1. _____	4. _____	◯
2. _____		
3. _____		

Workout Summary & Diet Notes:	TODAY'S GOALS	DONE?
Sleep Hours	1. _____	◯
	2. _____	◯
Daily Successes:	3. _____	◯
1. _____	4. _____	◯
2. _____		
3. _____		

FRIDAY

Day in review – What made today memorable?

SATURDAY

Day in review – What made today memorable?

SUNDAY

Day in review – What made today memorable?

Highlights of this Week

1. _____
2. _____
3. _____
4. _____
5. _____

Top Priorities For Next Week

1. _____ 4. _____
2. _____ 5. _____
3. _____ 6. _____

Weekly Summary (good/bad/other/weight/etc.)

Reminder From Your Past Self

Workout Summary & Diet Notes:

Sleep Hours

Daily Successes:

1.
2.
3.

TODAY'S GOALS

DONE?

1.
2.
3.
4.

Workout Summary & Diet Notes:

Sleep Hours

Daily Successes:

1.
2.
3.

TODAY'S GOALS

DONE?

1.
2.
3.
4.

Workout Summary & Diet Notes:

Sleep Hours

Daily Successes:

1.
2.
3.

TODAY'S GOALS

DONE?

1.
2.
3.
4.

Fitness Highlights of this Week

1.
2.
3.
4.
5.

Weekly Fitness Notes

RHR

BP

Total Distance
(in miles)

Week

Year

Weight

WEEK 52

Made in the USA
Coppell, TX
10 January 2021